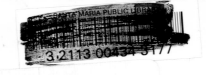

Everything

Women of Color

Should Know About

Cosmetic Surgery

Everything Women of Color Should Know About Cosmetic Surgery

Jan R. Adams, M.D.

ST. MARTIN'S PRESS ❦ NEW YORK

www.stmartins.com

Library of Congress Cataloging-in-Publication Data
Adams, Jan R.
  Everything women of color should know about cosmetic surgery/Jan R. Adams.
      p.   cm.
  ISBN 0-312-25310-9
  1. Surgery, Plastic.   2. Women—Surgery.   3. Afro-American women—Surgery. I. Title.

RD119 .A33 2000
617.9'5'089—dc21

                                              00-040241

First Edition: December 2000

10 9 8 7 6 5 4 3 2 1

A Note to Readers

This book is for informational purposes only. Readers are advised to consult a trained medical professional before acting on any of the information in this book.

In the following pages, the very intimate and personal feelings of some extraordinary individuals are presented to help you, the reader, understand the process of aesthetic plastic surgery.

The names used in the histories are fictitious and were chosen at random. The histories themselves represent compilations from a number of patients, and in no way correspond to any particular individual, nor are they indicative of any of the names used.

Likewise, the photos used were chosen to demonstrate important points about the procedures and in no way correspond to the names or the histories used in the text.

Thus, with the doctor–patient relationship intact, enjoy.

Contents

Introduction   ix

Part One: The Basics

1. Getting Started the Right Way   3
2. Choosing an Aesthetic Surgeon   14
3. Things to Do Before Surgery   23
4. Things to Expect Postoperatively   34
5. Scarring and Wound Healing   43
6. Skin Care   55

Part Two: The Twenties

7. Rhinoplasty (Nose Surgery)   75
8. Breast Augmentation   90
9. Reduction Mammoplasty   103

Part Three: The Thirties

10. Suction-Assisted Lipectomy   117
11. Mastopexy (Breast Lift)   133
12. Abdominoplasty (Tummy Tuck)   143

Part Four: The Forties

13. Browlift/Blepharoplasty (Eyes)   155

Part Five: **The Fifties**

14. Facelift   173

Part Six: **The Sixties and Beyond**

15. Touch-ups   191
16. The Successful Aging Beauty Solution   195

Introduction

THIS BOOK IS WRITTEN especially for women of color. It is a celebration of your beauty and diversity. It is also a practical guide to aesthetic surgery and what it can do to help you look and feel your best. Most important, this book is a blueprint for being healthy, vibrant, and youthful at any age. In these pages, we will discuss aesthetic surgical procedures that are specific to the particular issues that affect women of color, but we will also address issues concerning wellness, including nutrition, exercise, and skin care.

I was driven to write this book by my patients, many of whom experienced years of pain and frustration before they came to see me. They were suffering needlessly, unable to find either answers to their cosmetic problems or doctors sympathetic to their needs. I soon realized that information about their aesthetic surgery choices was not readily available. As amazing and appalling as it may seem, there isn't much information out there about aesthetic surgery for people of color. For much too long these patients—women of color—have been taken for granted. Their concerns about beauty, aging, skin care, and plastic surgery have been ignored by doctors, cosmetologists, and manufacturers of beauty products. So I decided to do something about it. I knew that with my patients' help, I could write a book that would empower you, the woman of color, and put an end to some of your pain and frustration.

As a black aesthetic plastic surgeon practicing in Beverly Hills, I am uniquely qualified to guide you through the ins and outs of being healthy and beautiful at any age. I worked long and hard to get where I am today. I graduated from Harvard University with honors. I attended the Ohio State University College of Medicine, where I received honors in all my major rotations. I trained in general surgery for five years at the Lenox Hill Hospital in Manhattan, where I

was chief resident in surgery in my final year. My plastic and reconstructive surgery training was at the University of Michigan in Ann
Arbor, where I also served as chief resident in plastic surgery. Then
UCLA offered me the first university-affiliated fellowship in aesthetic plastic surgery, and I jumped at the opportunity. I now have
sixteen years in aesthetic surgery from some of America's finest insti-
tutions.

My office is located on a block of Bedford Drive in Beverly Hills
that stretches between Little Santa Monica and Brighton Way. This
small geographic area houses at least fifty plastic surgeons. Beverly
Hills is the center of plastic surgery in California. After completion
of my training in plastic surgery, I had taken an associate position
with Dr. John Williams, the preeminent plastic surgeon in aesthetic
surgery, but after two years, I left to start my own practice. In order
to get to the next level as a plastic surgeon, I knew I had to go solo.

In a sense, I had to declare that I was the captain of the ship. Besides, it was important that I, as a black man, show the world that I
was performing surgery on a standard as high, if not higher, than the
next guy. I especially wanted my patients to know that they were
getting the best that plastic surgery had to offer. Second-class citi-
zenship is not good enough for me, and it certainly is not good
enough for my patients. By moving my office to Beverly Hills, I was
moving into the big leagues.

My office is in the older of two medical complexes in the neighbor-
hood. Most of the local plastic surgeons have offices in the shiny new
building on Bedford with its open, arched entryway that is three floors
high. The archway encircles a large, modern, brick-fronted building
with green trim. The elevators to the suites open onto the street, so
you don't even have to enter the building to use them. On the ground
floor are the fashionable boutiques that define Beverly Hills.

My building is not so monumental, though it is truly Beverly
Hills. The building is small and elegant, with a long history. The

walls are wood-paneled from floor to ceiling, and the bricks are real, not matted. The atmosphere is as warm and inviting as a grandparent's home. Patients—particularly older people—often say they used to see a doctor, now retired or perhaps passed away, who had an office in the building. The complex has inspired many memories for the people of Beverly Hills, and I certainly want it to house memories for me throughout a long and successful career. I chose to locate my practice in this building because it feels like it has been around forever, and I wanted everybody to know that I was here to stay.

For the last five years, I have been in private practice. That practice overwhelmingly involves women of color. I began as most plastic surgeons start out, first covering emergency rooms and hospitals, and then moving slowly into an aesthetic surgery practice that deals exclusively in elective cosmetic procedures. I perform hundreds of aesthetic procedures a year, including eyelid surgery, brow and face lifts, nose surgery, breast surgery, tummy tucks, and liposuction. I have performed over three thousand aesthetic surgery procedures, more than 80 percent of which have been performed on women of color.

Aesthetic surgery is becoming more and more popular among women of color. American women of color in fact, undergo more than 63,000 procedures annually. That represents a whopping $220,108,000 a year in elective surgery costs. It is certainly time someone gave you sound information about your surgical options. I can provide that information because of what I've learned as an aesthetic surgeon, not just from the medical school professors and other doctors, but from many of my remarkable patients.

This book features the stories of real women who have found their way to my office over the years. Many of their concerns are probably not much different from your own. They share personal struggles with beauty, aging, and self-worth that are, in many ways, universal. They also face problems such as scarring, skin blotchiness, and anxiety about the shape of their nose that are of specific relevance to you, women of color. You will experience their problems through their own eyes and hearts. Most important, you will come to understand the procedures that can solve these problems.

Inspired by my patients' desires to look and feel good, I have developed a lifetime plan for maintaining vitality and preserving youthful beauty. I am determined to help women of color age gracefully and with confidence. By following this plan, you can always look and feel great. The secret is simply to take good care of yourself, both mentally and spiritually, and address physical concerns with small, age-appropriate, rejuvenative surgical procedures. By doing so you can make that "done" look and the health risks that come from having a major surgical overhaul later in life, a thing of the past.

This strategy works because the changes that occur in our bodies with age happen in a common chronological pattern. These changes may become more diverse and variable with age, but by and large, we are all destined to experience them.

For example, in our thirties, most of us discover that those excess pounds and bulges that used to disappear with a jog around the block are suddenly harder to lose. In our forties, that tired look around the eyes greets us in the morning despite plenty of rest. My philosophy is to address these changes as they occur rather than waiting until they all overwhelm a woman in her sixties and then trying to fix everything at once. Rejuvenative plastic surgery should be used for maintenance rather than a makeover.

It is also important to take measures to prevent those modifiable aspects of aging that can be controlled. I will show you simple ways to establish good habits—a healthy diet, regular exercise, and a protective skin care regimen that will keep you beautiful inside and out, both physically and spiritually.

The book is designed to be a reference book. I realize that some women will want to read it straight through, while others will flip to the information relevant to their needs. As a result, the beginning of the book is devoted to general issues in aesthetic surgery, including choosing a surgeon, what to expect pre- and postoperatively, and how to establish a plan that is right for you and your needs. The rest of the book deals with specific procedures. We will discuss how to prepare yourself, the specific complications associated with each procedure, and with the questions you need to ask your surgeon before you agree to surgery.

It is my hope that however you decide to use this book, it inspires you to take control of your self-image, your aging process, and, ultimately, your life. Knowledge is power only if you use it. I wish you the best.

-Part One-

The Basics

Getting Started the Right Way

THE DECISION TO HAVE an elective cosmetic surgical procedure is never an easy one. There are so many difficult issues to deal with: the cost of the surgery, the fear of anesthesia, the anticipation of pain and discomfort, and the difficulty of discussing one's private wishes in a public forum with medical practitioners, family, and friends. This process, however, can be made much less stressful if you understand a few simple rules.

Rule #1: It's OK to Want to Look Your Best

There are many very sound reasons to have plastic surgery, though some people may tell you otherwise. I was recently asked to participate in a panel discussion o "Plastic Surgery for Women of Color" on a Los Angeles radio station. I thought I'd been recruited to discuss state-of-the-art cosmetic surgery as it pertained to minority women. But the host of the program neglected to tell me in advance that the subtitle of the debate was "A Manifestation of Self-Hate Imposed Upon Women of Color by a Racist Society." I nearly collapsed when I realized that the other panel members—a psychologist and a feminist activist—took the position that women, especially women of color, who have plastic surgery are engaged in self-mutilation because they don't like who they are. They went so far as to say, emphatically, that those women were actually trying to look white.

Now, this is an unsubstantiated, shallow argument that collapses under the weight of its own ignorance. Psychologists and psychiatrists, along with racial bigots on both sides of the fence, have often attempted to equate a woman's desire for physical improvement through cosmetic surgery with some psychopathologic condition akin to self-mutilation. There is no basis for this argument, except for the universal truth that most people make sacrifices in order to appear attractive and desirable. Adorning ourselves with paint, tattoos, scars, jewelry, unnatural hairstyles, or uncomfortable clothing dates from antiquity. Vanity, it would seem, is shared by all members of the human race despite our differences in sex, race, religion, and place of origin.

It's all very nice to say you shouldn't judge a book by its cover, that it is the content that's important. But that's not the way the world works. Appearance counts in all walks of life, from the cradle to the grave. Cute babies receive more attention; attractive children get better grades and more recognition from their teachers; good-looking employees command better jobs with higher salaries.

So let's put one issue to rest: *Women of color seeking plastic surgery consultation do not hate themselves and they are not trying to look white.* The overwhelming majority of my patients are indeed quite beautiful by any standard. They want to establish a balance in a feature that is incongruent with the rest of their body, or to address those inevitable changes that occur with aging.

Rule #2: *Understand Your Motives*

There are many legitimate and psychologically healthy reasons for you to consider having plastic surgery. If you want a nose job, that does not mean you hate yourself and wish you were white. Perhaps your nose is simply out of proportion with your other features and it will make you feel better about yourself to fix it. Still, regardless of the type of surgery you're interested in having done, it is important for you to understand your motivations and to make sure they're healthy ones.

As you begin to explore your surgical options, be prepared for people to question your motives—even your doctor. Do not take this to heart. Your doctor did not grow up or train for a plastic surgery career in a vacuum. Medical professionals can be subject to the same prejudices as everyone else. You can alleviate your doctor's fears or concerns by truthfully evaluating and answering some simple questions. I guarantee that your doctor will try to discover the answers to the following questions during your initial consultation, even if he or she doesn't ask them directly. If you can give honest, thoughtful answers, your consultation will go smoothly. Both you and your doctor will come away feeling informed and reassured.

- What results do I want to achieve? Are they reasonable?
- Can I be satisfied?
- Am I egocentric, overdemanding, or difficult to communicate with?
- Am I seeking cosmetic surgery for my own reasons or for someone else's?
- Is my significant other—my husband or boyfriend, wife or girlfriend—against my having this procedure?
- Am I willing to explore with a professional the relationship between my self-image and my desire to change my appearance?
- Would I be willing to undergo a psychiatric evaluation in an open, unbiased manner?
- Am I having marital problems, recently divorced, or undergoing a sudden change in job status?
- Have I recently lost a loved one?

For example, if you admit that you are seeking cosmetic surgery to please someone else rather than yourself, you should reconsider having the procedure done. If you really don't want it, why undergo the pain and expense of the surgery? It will not make you happy.

If a significant other is against it, you should also reconsider doing the procedure. You will certainly require the help of loved ones in the immediate postoperative period.

The point is that a positive answer to either of these questions is grounds to reconsider surgery. It does not mean that you should not have the procedure done, but it may mean that you are setting yourself up for failure because your reasons for having the surgery are not your own.

Your answers to all of these questions help your surgeon understand your reasons for seeking plastic surgery and will allow him to evaluate whether you're mentally prepared for the procedure. Knowing the answers to these questions *before* your arrival at the doctor's office will help you prepare for what is ahead of you. Please take some time to think about these issues. You may even want to discuss them with a friend or loved one before making a doctor's appointment. Knowing what you want and why you want it can only help you achieve your goals.

Rule #3: *Plastic Surgery Is a Tool—Make It Work for You*

When people talk about plastic surgery, they're usually referring to a specific branch of the discipline known as *aesthetic surgery*, which deals with aging and its cosmetic effects on appearance. In this book we will focus mainly on aesthetic surgery, the goal of which is to help you look as young as you feel. In this regard, the needs of women of color are no different from those of any other human being.

You may have said to yourself, "I feel young, I'm active, but I look in the mirror and I see a person who looks old to me. I want to do something about it." And so you should. A good plastic surgeon can help you recapture outwardly the person who still resides on the inside. The person who is energetic and fun. The person who loves life. The person who won't be repressed by babies, aging, or sun damage. A good plastic surgeon can help you be the person you want to be.

Aging is a hot topic these days. Everyone wants to live a long time, but no one wants to look or feel old. If I asked you if human beings are living longer, you would probably say yes. However, you would be wrong. We are not living longer. Don't feel bad, it's a trick question. When we talk about living longer, we have to distinguish between three different concepts: maximum life potential, the average life span, and life expectancy. Maximum life potential for human beings is somewhere around 120 years, and it has not changed for a thousand years. The average life span is approximately 85 to 90 years of age, and it also has not changed. Life expectancy, however, is another matter. Life expectancy—the number of years of life expected from birth—has been increasing. Today it's about 78 years of age, and that's certainly up from a hundred years ago.

What's interesting, however, is that as more people approach the average life span due to an increase in life expectancy, the age at which they begin to experience sickness also rises. Because life span is fixed, this means that the length of time between the onset of that sickness and death is decreasing. Simply put, it just means that older people in today's world are more vibrant and healthy, and that they are sick for a shorter time before they die. We can, however, age gracefully. We can find ways to avoid the complications of aging until the last possible moment. We can find ways to preserve our youth and vitality.

Let me explain how aesthetic surgery can help make this possible. We all know people of the same chronological age who have different physical or mental ages. Everyone has that aunt who is 50 but looks 35. That aunt may have a girlfriend who went to high school with her, but instead of looking 35 or even 50, she looks 70. The difference in these two women is variability. We age at different rates regardless of the markers we use to define aging. These differences get greater the older we get.

There is a reason for this variation in aging markers, other than pure chance. That reason is *plasticity.* Plasticity implies that there is a way to manipulate the different rates of maturing and exchange a rapid rate of aging for a slower rate. The secret is to identify those markers of aging that can be changed and manipulate them. Some markers can be easily modified. For example, the body tends to get flabby with age, but regular exercise can give a 50-year-old woman the same muscle tone as a 20-year-old. Other age markers, like wrinkles around the eyes or sagging breasts, can't be remedied so easily. For those, rejuvenative surgery can help turn back the clock.

Rule #4: Don't Wait Until You Hate the Face in the Mirror

We know what changes to expect in our appearance as we age. We also know approximately at what stage—or age—these changes will occur. By planning ahead, it is possible to control the timing and the cost of plastic surgery procedures. My advice is to start fighting the aging process *before* you hate that face in the mirror. Otherwise, you'll end up wanting a massive makeover when you're older. Having major work done all at once is never a good idea. It's hard on your body and rarely looks natural. In fact, it can leave you looking like you're constantly startled or surprised. Instead, use smaller procedures earlier in life for maintenance. They cost less in terms of both money and recovery time.

In general, different aesthetic surgical procedures are appropriate at different times of life. Below is a general guideline for deciding at what age to consider addressing certain problems. I will discuss these procedures further in later chapters.

- *The Twenties:* Most women in their twenties are concerned about form rather than aging or gravity. Procedures such as *rhinoplasty* (nose surgery), *breast augmentation,* and *breast reduction,* make sense for women in this age group.
- *The Thirties:* Women in their thirties, particularly if they have finished childbearing, want to recapture their youthful figures. Exercise alone may not do the trick. Slowing of the body's metabolism and the effects of childbearing are the culprits here. Women who have lost breast volume or have breast ptosis (drooping) can benefit from *mastopexy* (a breast lift). *Liposuction* can help improve the appearance of flabby areas that do not respond to exercise. For women who have a complete loss of the integrity of the abdominal wall and stretch marks due to childbearing, a *tummy tuck* may be the answer.
- *The Forties:* Women usually start to see signs of aging in the face by their early forties. Often this takes the form of fine wrinkles around the eyes and a drooping of the brow. In a few unfortunate individuals, this can manifest as jowling of the cheeks or wrinkling of the skin of the neck. For women of color, this period is characterized mainly by brow and eyelid changes. The most beneficial procedure for these problems is a *brow lift* or *blepharoplasty,* which is eyelid surgery. Many women in their forties also consider body contour procedures like *liposuction* if they haven't already been addressed.
- *The Fifties:* The early fifties is often the time to consider a *facelift* procedure. That's because the effects of gravity begin to show on the lower face. The good news is that many women of color don't need this procedure. You don't show

age in the lower face at the same rate that Caucasian women often do.

· ***The Sixties:*** If you've taken good care of yourself and used surgery as maintenance rather than a makeover, you may not need any more surgery. The most you'll have to consider is a minor touch-up. This is good news because now is not the best time to bear the cost or the trauma of multiple procedures done simultaneously in a desperate attempt to regain some youthfulness. Also, you won't have to worry about having that "done" look that comes from doing everything at once.

Rule #5: *Protect Your Assets*

Plastic surgery is a powerful tool that will help you age beautifully, but it needs to be used in conjunction with eating right, exercise, and good skin and hair care. For the best long-term beauty results, you need to learn to take care of your assets. Here are some easy tips on how to keep your body beautiful.

NUTRITION

Eating right is of paramount importance. I recommend a see-food diet. If you see food, eat it. I want you to win. Life is hard enough without denying yourself the things you like. There are, however, some things you can do to improve your eating habits and your overall health.

· ***Eat Less.*** Eat everything you like, just less of it. Try to limit the number of calories you take in to less than 1,500 kilocalories per day. That's it. You don't have to compulsively count calories or deny yourself what you like. Just rethink how you go about it. For example, if you like Big Macs, eat them. I know, none of us admit to eating at McDonald's, but if you do, instead of ordering two Big Macs and supersizing it, order just one and have a small order of fries. Drink water instead of Coke. Right there you've done something you enjoy, and at the same time you've reduced your caloric intake by about half. You can do the same thing at Grandma's house, too. I know you don't want to offend her by not eating, but if you lose weight she won't talk about you to your cousins when you and the kids have gone home.

· *Minimize your intake of fried foods, vegetable oils, and salad dressings.* These contain oils, which result in the production of free radicals. Free radicals are groups of elements or atoms that carry an unpaired electron and no charge. They are thought to be a factor in cell injury and aging. Many diseases, including some cancers, may be the result of free radical injury to cells.

· *Try to decrease the amount of sugar in your diet.* I don't want to suggest that sugar is bad in and of itself. Your brain and muscles use sugar to produce energy. However, sugar can increase mineral loss from the body by increasing urine output.

· *Take dietary supplements as part of your daily routine in order to ensure that your body gets the building blocks it needs.* These supplements should include minerals and trace elements, vitamins, essential amino acids, and essential fatty acids.

SKIN CARE

Most women, and nearly all men, don't focus on skin care until they have problems. These problems include wrinkles, dark spots, and even cancer. Remember this: *The best way to treat a disease is not with medications and surgery; the best way to treat a disease is never to get it.* The sun is the number one cause of premature skin aging. Unfortunately, many people, particularly women of color, are under the misguided impression that if you have dark skin, you're protected from the harmful effects of the sun. The truth is that dark-skinned people have more natural protection than fair-skinned people, but the sun can still cause damage. The best protection is complete avoidance of the sun, but this is hardly feasible. The solution is sun protection, and that means a sunblock. I don't want to give you a sense of false security with that, either. Sunblock provides limited protection. I also realize that it is difficult to get women of color to wear sunblock. Most of these medications go on chalky white and give the skin an ashen look, that sort of grayish hue to the skin that you see on a corpse.

There is, however, a solution. I have developed a moisturizer with sunblock and antioxidants that's specifically for use on dark skin. The product contains melanin, a natural sunblock, instead of acetyl methoxycyrinate, to prevent that ashen look. Melanin offers similar sun protection without the grayish hue. Rudalgo Solutions, my skin care line, also includes facial cleansers, non-soap bar cleansers, and body moisturizers, which contain state-of-the-art ingredients. Whatever products you use, is it important to start with smart skin care now. It can help you avoid problems in the future.

In particular, you can avoid some of those unsolvable problems that women of color present within their forties and fifties. These include *blotchiness* and hyperpigmentation.

More information about these products can be obtained by writing to:

J Rudalgo Skin Care, Inc.
P.O. Box 5888
Beverly Hills, CA 90209-5888

EXERCISE

Do not underestimate the importance of exercise. It's essential to keep your body in shape. Our society puts so much emphasis on youth and adolescent sports programs, yet exercise is even more beneficial to people over thirty. That's when your body begins to deteriorate rather than grow. After thirty, your body slows down and you lose flexibility. Exercise is the key to maintaining muscle mass, losing excess fat, and staying flexible. You *must* develop a personalized exercise program. Be realistic and choose a plan you can stick with. Here are some factors to consider:

- The best time to discover activities you enjoy is in your youth. Kids play and exercise all the time. Think back to what sports you enjoyed as a child.
- Try to find an activity that you can do for the rest of your life. Learn to play tennis or golf or simply get hooked on aerobics or walking.
- Consider sports that you can do by yourself or with one person. Organized sports are great when you are young, but if your activity requires getting ten adults together who all have careers and families, it will never happen.
- Choose something that you can do every day.

If you're willing to take these small steps to improve your health and appearance, you'll find that you feel better about yourself. The confidence that comes from liking yourself will be your greatest asset. Indeed, it will help you in every aspect of your life.

2

Choosing an Aesthetic Surgeon

FINDING THE RIGHT SURGEON takes time. It requires some general knowledge and a little research. This chapter will tell you everything you need to know in order to find the best possible physician to perform your procedure. You'll learn what to look for in a surgeon, what to avoid, and the questions to ask to make sure a doctor is right for you.

To begin with, you need to understand the difference between the four major plastic surgery specialties:

- *Cranial-facial surgery.* This specialty deals with bones in the face. These doctors do most of their work on pediatric patients and accident victims.
- *Reconstructive surgery.* This specialty involves moving muscle flaps and tissue to close wounds.
- *Hand surgery.* As you'd expect, these doctors specialize in treating the problems of the bones, muscles, and tissues of the hand.
- *Aesthetic surgery, or cosmetic surgery.* This is the specialty that most of us are referring to when we talk about plastic surgery. These surgeons specialize in cosmetic procedures that combat the effects of aging on appearance.

Chances are, the right doctor for you is an aesthetic surgeon. We've narrowed the field a bit, but there's a long way to go. For starters, there are countless aesthetic surgeons. And there are many doctors from other specialties performing cosmetic procedures. One reason so many different specialists are now performing plastic surgery has to do with health care reform.

The rise of managed care has caused many doctors' revenues to shrink considerably over the past few years. As revenues have dropped, outside specialists have entered the cosmetic surgery arena hoping to make up that lost income. Gynecologists have begun doing suction-assisted lipectomy, commonly known as liposuction. Dermatologists are doing facelifts. Oral surgeons are starting to include rhino-plasty—nose surgery—in their repertoire. And otolaryngologists, or ear, nose, and throat doctors, are promoting themselves as facial plastic surgeons. In short, the competition for the cosmetic surgery patient, which until recently was solely the domain of the plastic surgeon, has increased considerably. In the long run, this will benefit patients. Competition will mean lower prices and improved techniques.

But right now the competition and confusion mean that patients have to be more careful than ever about choosing a doctor. Some of the doctors doing cosmetic surgeries are performing them in outpatient clinics rather than hospitals. They're also forming different medical societies and boards. As a physician, I myself can't keep these people straight. It is no wonder the public is confused. It can be extremely difficult to tell which doctors are adequately trained to do what procedures. Here are a few general guidelines to ensure that your doctor is qualified to perform aesthetic surgery:

· Get a list of the reputable surgeons in your area who perform the surgery you want. If you go to the state medical board, they will direct you to the licensing organization. This is a good place to start, but it does not guarantee that you will find the right doctor. Just because a physician is licensed, and just because he's boarded in some specialty, doesn't mean he has the expertise or the experience in the procedure you want. Board certification means that a physician has fulfilled the requirements, including years of training, a generalized written exam, and an oral exam in his specialty within a specified time.

· Choose a trained aesthetic surgeon rather than someone who's expertise is in a completely different area. Also, make certain that your surgeon can address all possible complications. You want someone who can fix problems and did not simply learn to do a procedure.

· If you choose a surgeon from another specialty, make sure he or she has training in more than just one way to solve your problem. Your doctor should be able to give you a number of alternatives.

· Choose a doctor affiliated with a hospital. Hospitals require credentialing based on a surgeon's training. If your physician is not credentialed to do an operation in a hospital, he probably should not be doing it in a surgicenter. A surgicenter is a freestanding operating room separate from the hospital. These facilities are required to meet the same specifications as a hospital operating room.

Once you have a list of qualified doctors in your area, it's time to narrow it down. It doesn't make sense to meet with every doctor on the list. You don't want to waste the doctor's time, and, most importantly, you don't want to waste your time and money. I once met a woman who felt it was a badge of honor that she had had consultations with sixteen doctors before deciding on a surgeon. That's crazy! Why would you go to sixteen doctors' offices asking them the same thing? I'm all for getting adequate information, but sixteen different opinions on the same question can only serve to confuse you.

Instead of making a bunch of consultation appointments, do some research and narrow down the list to your top one or two choices. You can always consult with a third doctor if the first two don't work out. Here are a few ways to shorten the list:

- *Know what you want in a doctor.* I have had women make appointments, come in and talk for two hours, and then tell a friend, "I liked what he said but I wouldn't go to a black doctor.' They knew I was black before they got there, so what's the point? If it's important to you that your doctor is a woman, or is a Harvard Medical School graduate, or is affiliated with a certain hospital, that's fine. Consult with doctors who meet your criteria and don't waste anyone else's time.
- *Ask friends for recommendations.* Ask everyone you know if they have a good surgeon. Your best sources will be people who have had the procedure you're interested in. If they liked their doctor, check to see if he's on your list of qualified surgeons. If he's not, consider adding him to your list. A recommendation from someone you trust is a good sign that a doctor is adequate for your needs.
- *Choose a doctor who makes you comfortable.* In addition to being qualified, your plastic surgeon should be someone who makes you feel at ease. Ask around and find out what kind of personality a potential surgeon has. This is an important factor. You want to have a rapport with your doctor. Perhaps you feel best when your doctor is very businesslike, or maybe you prefer someone more informal. Only you can decide what type of person makes you most comfortable.

The Consultation

Now that you've done your homework, make appointments with the doctor or doctors you have chosen. Give the receptionist your name, age, and the procedure or problem for which you are seeking consultation. She will want your telephone number and your address in the event that they need to send you information prior to your consultation. The doctor may also request a consultation fee. I generally don't request a fee if a patient is referred by one of my other patients. However, if it's a second opinion, I charge a fee that ranges from $150 to $300. For those new patients seeking information, the fee is $250 and is applied to the cost of surgery once the procedure is scheduled. These days, with the intense competition for patients, some doctors don't charge this fee. I would advise you not to take a doctor off your list just because he charges a consulting fee. Remember, that money generally can be applied toward the cost of your surgery. And if you've done your research, chances are you're consulting with the right doctor for you. Understand that a surgeon can't stay in business if he spends all his time giving advice to people who are simply window-shopping.

BE PREPARED

Before your appointment, make a written list of all the questions you have for the doctor. This ensures that you won't forget anything and that all your concerns will be addressed by the doctor. We will discuss the types of questions you may want to ask later in this chapter.

ARRIVE EARLY FOR YOUR APPOINTMENT

You're going to have medical forms to fill out. Get this out of the way so you have more time with the doctor. The paperwork generally consists of a patient identification form, a health questionnaire, insurance verification forms, a request for general information about the problem for which you have scheduled the consultation, and a physician–patient arbitration agreement.

The physician–patient arbitration agreement is a legal document By signing the physician-patient arbitration agreement, *both parties* are entering into a contract whereby any dispute as to medical malpractice is determined by arbitration rather than in a court of law before a jury. The agreement can be revoked by written notice delivered to the physician within thirty days of signature. It creates a certain amount of dissonance for both the patient and the doctor. I can tell you from the doctor's point of view that before I meet somebody and have an opportunity to discuss their problems, I don't want to start talking about what can go wrong. In my mind, the doctor must be the patient advocate. The arbitration agreement generally presents itself as a hindrance to establishing a healthy doctor–patient relationship. That's unfortunate, because good communication between the doctor and the patient is important to getting good results. Understand that in today's society, this form is a necessary evil. It's up to your discretion whether you sign the arbitration form or not. You may want to talk to the doctor, get a feel for him, and then choose whether or not to sign the agreement after your consultation. It's really up to you.

MEETING THE DOCTOR

The consultation itself can take many forms. It depends on the surgeon. I prefer to meet a patient in my private office rather than an exam room. I want to meet you in a situation that is relaxed. That way, should your exam require that you remove any clothing, you will have had an opportunity to get comfortable. I know I'd prefer to meet someone before I disrobed in front of them. It also gives me an opportunity to explain the procedure clearly, without distractions, while both of us are focused.

When we first get together, I try to learn a little bit about who you are, your marital status, how many children you have, what you do for a living, previous surgeries, transportation to and from the surgical center, and whether your family knows about the proposed surgery. My thoroughness is to ensure safety. I want to make sure that everyone is on the same page and that you have a safe, pleasant experience.

After we've discussed your medical history, we will turn to your main reason for the consultation. You're given the opportunity to spell out in no uncertain terms what you would like. I ask—in fact, I demand—that you be specific. *You must be clear about what you want.* One of the saddest things in plastic surgery is the patient who is unhappy with a very good result. More often than not, it's due to a breakdown in communication. The patient went to a plastic surgeon to get her nose fixed, for example. She wasn't clear about what she wanted. As a result, the surgeon wasn't able to translate her desires into something anatomic. The patient didn't get what she had hoped for, and the surgeon wasn't in a position to perform his best work because he wasn't clear about the goal either. This is a disaster for both of them.

Everyone is different. The surgeon must design a procedure that best solves your individual problem. Avoid surgeons who do an operation only one way regardless of the patient. If the doctor says, "This is how I do it," you should head for the door. You, the patient, and your body type should determine how a physician carries out a procedure. Ask the surgeon for alternatives, and the other types of methods to solve your specific problem.

THE EXAM

After we finish discussing the procedures designed to solve your problem, we then go to the exam room. Here we talk about specifics.

Together we will design a procedure that is best for you. The examination may require that you disrobe. If it does, I will allow you time to disrobe alone and get dressed in private. Some physicians will ask a nurse to accompany him at this time for medical-legal reasons. This is certainly reasonable and is done to ensure your welfare.

When the exam is finished, we will continue the consultation back in my office with you fully dressed and comfortable again. I, for one, don't think it's fair to engage you in a long conversation while I stand there fully clothed and you're nude. That will only make you feel more insecure. I want to level the playing field as much as possible so that you feel confident in expressing what you want. If you are clear about what you want, it makes my job much easier and a lot more fun.

ASKING QUESTIONS

Now is the time to ask any questions that have not been answered. The kinds of questions you ask will depend on what you're looking for. You can get specific about the proposed incisions and the expected result. Most physicians will discuss the risks, benefits, and possible complications of surgery at this time. Any physician not willing to discuss these types of issues should be avoided. If it hasn't been covered, ask about the postoperative course and follow-up exams. I generally see people one to two days after the surgery to make sure things are OK and then five to seven days after surgery to remove sutures. At three weeks after surgery, I will see you in order to get you back to your regular activity. Other follow-up visits are determined by the procedures performed.

The final issue to be addressed at the initial examination is the cost of the surgery. Don't be bashful. Ask it straight up. It's your money you're spending, and you should know how much it is going to cost.

THE PREOPERATIVE EXAM

If you are interested in going ahead with the surgery, we will schedule a preoperative examination. This second visit gives you time to go home and digest what is said at our first meeting. It also allows you time to think of other questions or issues you may need clarified prior to surgery. Avoid those surgeons who pressure you to commit to surgery immediately. You, after all, are the important person in this interaction, and the doctor and his staff are there to serve you.

The second preoperative exam is scheduled for three weeks prior to your surgery date. In my mind, these two meetings together constitute the consultation. The initial consultation fee therefore covers this visit. At this time, blood is drawn for laboratory examinations, preoperative photos are taken, and payment is due. I will give you a plastic surgery checklist to help guide you through the pre- and postoperative periods.

If you feel that your surgeon has been negligent in providing you with any information about your procedure, take the time to ask. The most important thing you can take away from your consultation is confidence in your doctor. And you'll feel assured only if he answers *all* your questions. Don't feel stupid about asking a "dumb" question. Surgery is a big deal. You need to be comfortable that this doctor can perform your procedure the way you want it done. Having a good working relationship with your physician is the best way to make sure your surgery is a complete success.

3

Things to Do Before Surgery

THE PERIOD THREE WEEKS prior to surgery is the most difficult. You will worry about everything from the anesthesia to the size of the incisions to the amount of time it will take you to recover. You will begin to question your motives. You may even begin to question whether you should be having surgery at all. This is all very natural and is part of the stress that accompanies elective surgery.

There are, however, a number of things you can do to make this period more tolerable.

Schedule the Preoperative Visit

Write down the date and time of your appointment for your reference. Make a list of information you want to receive from your doctor and questions you want answered during this consultation. Your list should include:

- Confirm the type of surgery you are having.
- Confirm the name and location of the hospital or surgical facility where your surgery will take place.
- Find out your expected time of arrival to the surgery center or hospital.
- Get a list of pre- and postoperative instructions and make sure you understand them all thoroughly.
- Any residual questions about your procedure you want answered should be answered now.

· Obtain prescriptions for postoperative medications, and fill them prior to surgery so they will be available afterward. (There is nothing worse than discovering once you are home and settled that you have no pain medication.)

During this appointment, your past medical history will be reviewed and any areas that require further attention will be addressed. Most people who choose to have cosmetic surgery are in excellent health, so this thorough investigation of your medical history may seem like overkill. But it is important to be safe. The best way to address problems and complications is to never develop them. In order to ensure that your body is prepared to undergo surgery, your doctor will perform some routine medical tests, or ask you to schedule them with your regular physician. Here are some of the tests that may be required before your surgery.

· *A general physical examination.* This is to ensure that you are in good health and that there is no medical reason why you shouldn't undergo surgery.

· *The Coulter blood count.* This test evaluates the status of your blood. It is especially helpful in detecting anemia.

· *Urinalysis.* This helps evaluate urinary tract infections and kidney abnormalities. An electrolyte evaluation and/or liver function test may also be obtained, although these are not routine.

· *Mammogram.* Women over the age of forty who are having breast surgery must have a mammogram if they haven't had one in the last year. Patients having breast augmentation should also have a mammogram approximately three months after the procedure. This serves as the baseline exam, giving radiologists who will evaluate future mammograms a point of reference. He or she will then be able to monitor any lesions that are suspicious or suggestive of cancer.

· *Electrocardiogram and chest x-ray.* Every patient over fifty, in addition to a complete physical examination, should arrange to have an electrocardiogram and a chest X ray. The electrocardiogram will be evaluated prior to surgery by a cardiologist, and a radiologist will examine the chest X ray.

· *Eye exam.* Patients having eyelid surgery who have not had a complete eye examination in the past year should do so. Insurance companies will not consider reimbursement for eligible eyelid procedures unless an eye doctor has performed a visual field study. Those who wear contact lenses should be aware that contacts should not be worn for five to seven days after eyelid surgery. Comfortably fitting glasses should be worn during this period.

In addition to these tests, you should be aware that many insurance carriers who allow reimbursement for certain procedures such as nasal septal surgery, upper eyelid surgery, breast reduction, and scar revision surgery may require second surgical opinions. Some carriers will give you the names of physicians within their network who are available for this purpose. It is your responsibility to check with your carrier. Understand that failure to obtain a required second opinion may decrease or eliminate any insurance rebate.

Avoid These Substances Before Surgery

There are many substances that can affect your health and ability to recover from your surgery. Your doctor may give you a list of what drugs you should avoid, but here are some general no-nos.

ASPIRIN

Two weeks before your surgery, you must give up all aspirin and aspirin-containing products. Aspirin prevents platelets from clumping together to form tissue plugs. Platelets are the blood products that help to seal wounds after an injury. Aspirin-containing products will increase bleeding and bruising. If you are taking any anti-inflammatory medication and are uncomfortable without it, your doctor can provide you with an aspirin-free substitute. For pain, take acetaminophen, such as Tylenol, instead of aspirin. The following table lists aspirin-containing drugs that must be discontinued two weeks prior to surgery. Two weeks following surgery, you may return to your regular aspirin-containing medications.

RECREATIONAL DRUGS

Even a small amount of marijuana, cocaine, or other drugs can have an impact on anesthesia and your subsequent healing. Stop using all of these drugs at least two weeks before surgery. Stopping altogether will certainly improve your health.

ALCOHOL

Abstain from all alcoholic beverages for at least two weeks before your surgery because alcohol provides calories without providing essential nutrients. This not only decreases appetite, but also causes

Table 1: Aspirin-containing medications. This is the short list of medications that contain aspirin. Aspirin inhibits platelet functions and can result in bleeding postoperatively. Always check with your physician and alert him or her to whatever medications you are taking. Ideally, these should be avoided for two weeks before and two weeks after surgery.

A.P.C.	Ecotrin
A.S.A. Compound	Empirin
Advil	Emprazil
Alka-Seltzer	Equagesic
Anacin	Exedrin
Anaprox	Feldene
Arthritis Pain Formula	Fiorinal
Ascodeen-30	Indocin
Ascriptin	Liquiprin Tablets
Aspergum	Midol
Aspirin	Measurin
Aspirin Suppositories	Monacet with Codeine
Bayer Aspirin Tablets	Motrin
Buff-A-Comp	Naprosyn
Buffadyn	Norgesic
Bufferin	Nuprin
Butabital	Pabrin Buffered Tab
Cama	PAC
Cheracol Capsules	Panalgesic
Clinoril	Percodan
Congespirin	Persistin
Copron Capsules	Phensol
Cope	Robaxisal
Coricidin C	Sodium Salicilate
Coumadin	Supac
Counter Pain	Tolectin
Darvon Compound	Triaminicin
Defort-Deful	Trigesic
Dolor	Vanquish
Dristan	Zomax
Duragesic	

You may return to your regular aspirin-containing medication schedule two weeks after surgery unless instructed otherwise.

RECREATIONAL OR SOCIAL DRUG USE:

Even a small amount of marijuana, cocaine, or other drugs can have an impact on your anesthesia and healing. Please stop completely at this time. Stopping altogether would markedly improve your health and extend your life.

malabsorption of nutrients through alcohol's toxic effects on the bowels and pancreas. In a sense, alcohol promotes malnutrition by interfering with the metabolism of carbohydrates and lipids. This malnutrition can adversely affect wound healing.

COFFEE, TEA, AND SODA

The caffeine in coffee, tea, and soda can be harmful because caffeine increases the urinary loss of calcium, magnesium, chloride, and potassium. It also can raise blood pressure significantly. Avoid drinking caffeinated beverages for two weeks before your surgery.

CIGARETTES

Cigarettes are bad for your health in general, but they are particularly harmful before surgery. The nicotine in cigarettes causes an increase in heart rate, an increase in blood pressure, and constriction of blood vessels in the skin, which can be disastrous in procedures such as a facelift. The constriction of the blood vessels decreases the flow of blood to the skin and can affect healing. Don't smoke for at least two weeks before your operation.

Practice Presurgery Hygiene

Three days before your operation, you should start taking some extra care with personal hygiene. Again, this may seem like overkill, but it is in your best interest to do everything possible to prevent complications. Here are some easy hygienic precautions that will lower your risk of infection.

- *Use antibacterial soap.* Begin showering daily with an antibacterial soap such as Phisoderm, Dial, or Zest.
- *Clean your ears.* If you are having facial or scalp surgery, gently clean out the crevices around and inside your ears with

a cotton-tip applicator. If you have a large quantity of wax build-up in your ears, eliminate it with either Diburox ear wax remover or Murine to prevent bacterial growth.

- **Don't shave under your arms.** This precaution is only necessary if you are having breast surgery. By not shaving your underarms for at least three days prior to surgery, you decrease the likelihood of postoperative infection.
- **Don't color your hair.** Avoid any kind of tinting, dyeing, or bleaching of your hair for at least three days prior to surgery. These processes can result in contact dermatitis of the skin. The inflammation can be characterized by redness, swelling, edema, crusting, scaling, and vesicles. Scratching or rubbing can lead to further problems, with the attendant possibility of increasing the likelihood of infection.

Get Organized

You'll feel less stressed about your surgery and recovery if you've tied up as many loose ends as possible before the procedure. This includes making sure things are covered at work and at home while you're out of commission. Here are a few details to remember:

- **Transportation.** Confirm transportation arrangements a week before surgery. Make sure everyone involved knows the location of the facility where your surgery will be performed.
- **Postop care.** Coordinate with the family member or friend who will be caring for you postoperatively. Have them read over your postoperative checklist and make sure they understand the procedures and instructions.
- **Prepare your recovery zone.** Remember that you won't be up to rearranging furniture or digging through cabinets looking for things immediately after your operation. Have

everything you may need conveniently located. For example, it may be beneficial to place a small stool in your shower. Early in your recovery, you may need to sit down when you bathe.

Twenty-Four Hours Before Surgery

At this point, you should be as prepared as possible for your surgery. Now is the time to relax and mentally prepare yourself for what's ahead. Don't worry if you're still a bit nervous. Focus on the beautiful results your surgery will soon yield. As you make final preparations for your big day, here are a few things to keep in mind.

- *Decide what to wear.* On the evening prior to surgery, set out your clothes for the next morning. Choose something loose that buttons or zips in the front. A warm jogging suit is ideal. Wear flat shoes that are easy to get on and off. Bring an extra pair of underpants. It is not necessary to wear pantyhose or a girdle. If you are going to a hospital or staying overnight in an outpatient facility, bring a bathrobe, pajamas or nightgown, slippers, toothpaste and toothbrush, a comb or brush, deodorant, and your prescription medication.
- *Do not wear makeup to the surgery center.* Your face (and the rest of you) should be clean for the surgery.
- *Don't style your hair.* Simply wash your hair with a mild shampoo the night before.
- *Don't wear jewelry, earrings, rings, hairpins, or false eyelashes.* These items get in the surgeon's way and must be removed. To avoid loss, keep them at home.
- *Wigs must be removed during surgery.* Patients who wear wigs should notify the nurse at the surgical facility. The wig will be removed before the surgery.

· *Bring eyeglasses, contacts, or dentures in their case.* These items cannot be worn during the surgery. Be sure your name is on the outside of the case so that they can be easily returned to you after your procedure.

· *Don't eat for at least six hours before surgery.* Your stomach must be empty when you are given anesthesia to help decrease nausea and avoid complications. Have a light meal the night before your surgery. Ideally, eat something high in protein like chicken or fish. If you are having surgery in the morning, do not eat or drink anything after midnight. People with severe medical problems, however, may take their regular prescription medications with a small sip of water. If your surgery is in the afternoon, you may have a clear liquid breakfast that morning.

· *Talk to the anesthesiologist.* If you are having general anesthesia, you will talk to the anesthesiologist on the night before your surgery and again in the morning. For many of you, undergoing anesthesia is your biggest fear. He will answer your questions and try to calm your anxieties. You will also discuss any prescription drugs you may be taking to make sure there will be no interactions with the anesthesia. Many people have trouble sleeping prior to surgery. The anesthesiologist can tell you what sleeping aids may be taken the night before.

The Big Day

On the morning of the surgery, you will feel quite anxious. If you didn't, I would think there was something wrong with you. The anxiety you feel is quite normal and will rapidly disappear once you have reached the surgery facility. Here's what to expect when you arrive.

· *Admission.* When you arrive, the nurses will admit you and get your appropriate medical information. Don't get upset if you are asked the same medical history questions by several different people. Understand that double- or even triple-checking is important for your safety. You will also be asked to sign a standard surgical consent form.

· *Meet with the anesthesiologist.* You will be familiar with the anesthesiologist having already met him or her prior to the procedure. Modern anesthesia techniques are extremely safe and comfortable. However, feel free to ask the anesthesiologist any questions or share any concerns that you may have with him. The anesthesiologist will be happy to talk with you about the procedure and about what will take place during the time you are asleep. He may or may not give you a mild sedative for relaxation.

· *Meet with the surgeon.* You will also see your doctor before you go into surgery. You will again discuss your planned

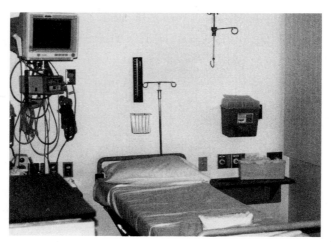

Figure 1: The preoperative holding area. Here you will be admitted to the surgery center. The nurses will help you change to a surgical gown and store your belongings, and you will have an opportunity to meet with the anesthesiologist.

procedure, and do whatever preoperative markings are appropriate. Additional preop photographs may be taken at this time. The doctor will answer any remaining questions that you may have.

After all the preliminaries have been taken care of, you will be taken to the operating room. There, you will be closely monitored by modern, computerized, state-of-the-art equipment. An intravenous line will be started by the anesthesiologist, and you will fall gently to sleep.

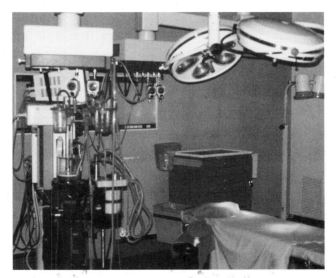

Figure 2: The operating room. There are many electronic monitoring devices within an operating room, and upon initial entry these gadgets can be quite intimidating.

4

Things to Expect Postoperatively

CONGRATULATIONS! YOU MADE IT. You survived the procedure! I knew you would, even though there were times you thought you wouldn't. You held your ground and did something for *you*. You thought carefully about the changes you wanted to make. You researched your options. You obtained opinions from qualified practitioners. And you followed through. I know it was difficult, and I applaud your courage.

Now that the hard part is over, you can breathe a sigh of relief and relax. In fact, you don't have a choice: You must take it easy for the next three weeks in order to let your body heal. It won't take three weeks for you to feel better, but you should give it at least that long before resuming all your normal activities.

The surgery is over, but the healing process itself can be challenging and emotionally traumatic. There will be physical pain to deal with. And you may even experience some sense of depression. It is perfectly normal. Just remember that it will soon pass and you'll be left with the results that you wanted in the first place.

What to Expect Immediately After Surgery

After surgery you'll be taken from the operating room to the recovery room. An oxygen mask will be lightly applied to your face to assist oxygenation. Oxygenation refers to enriching the blood with oxygen that can then be delivered to the body's tissues. You will be covered with a blanket for warmth. A blood pressure cuff, or sphyg-momanometer, will be placed on your upper arm. This cuff will become tight periodically as it takes your blood pressure. A small plastic finger clip, a pulse oximeter, will be attached to one of your fingers. This scans your blood to make certain you are getting adequate oxygen. There will be EKG leads on your chest to record your heart activity. All of this will create a constant beeping around you that is totally annoying. Try to ignore it. Most likely, you'll be too drugged to care and you really won't remember anyway.

Occasionally patients feel cold following surgery. It is not the room that is cold but rather the patient's body temperature, which has dropped during anesthesia. Blankets will be supplied to help keep you warm until your temperature returns to normal.

What you will probably remember is the annoying person working around your bed. You may be tempted to call her a witch, but she's the recovery room nurse and all the poking and prodding she's doing is for your own good. She's a doll, so be nice to her. You need her.

The First Few Days After Surgery

Once you fully regain consciousness, you're officially on the road to recovery. Here's what you need to know to get through those first few days after surgery.

· **Being tired is normal.** Immediately following surgery, your mind may be active, but your body will want to rest. Modern-day anesthetics leave your system fairly quickly, but for a day or two it is not unusual to feel tired or dizzy. This is complicated by pain medications that make you even more drowsy and uncoordinated. Don't fight it. Lie down when you feel like it. Your body needs sleep. This is all very normal.

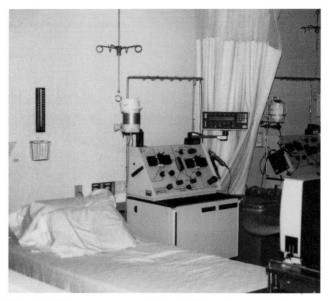

Figure 3: The recovery room. Quite similar to the preoperative holding area, the rtecovery room contains sophisticated monitoring machines and can be quite noisy.

- *Being anxious or nervous is normal.* You thought you would be relieved, and trust me, you will be! But feelings of anxiety, nervousness, and concern are all normal immediately following surgery. They will diminish rapidly as your recovery progresses. Try not to make the people around you crazy, especially the doctor. Relax and understand that this will all pass. Remember, the hard part is over.

- *Make yourself walk around.* Having surgery is not an excuse to lie in bed like a beached whale. When the effects of anesthesia have worn off and you are completely awake, get out of bed and walk around the room *with assistance.* One of the most feared complications of any surgery is a pulmonary embolism. That's a blood clot in a blood vessel in the lungs. It occurs because of immobilization and causes breathing difficulties and even death. Simply getting out of bed is the best way to prevent it from happening. If you can't walk, or simply refuse to, then change positions in bed. Move your legs and flex your ankles. Remember, being sedentary can kill you, so get up. Get up now!

· **Breathe deeply.** Your doctor has given you medication to help with the pain, and you're going to need it. Pain can prevent you from taking deep breaths. Don't wait until the pain is unbearable to take your pills. You'll be playing catch-up and never get any relief. It may be better to take them every three hours by the clock the first day. Take them as needed thereafter.

· **Take your antibiotics.** Your doctor may also have given you antibiotics to take. Take them until they are gone. You won't need any more, so don't ask for them.

· **Drink fluids.** You will probably be thirsty for the first few days, so drink plenty of fluids. Your thirst is caused by blood loss and fluid shifts within the body. Your body fluids should be back in alignment within three to five days. When that happens, you will have to urinate frequently.

· **Eat what you want.** For the first day or two after recovery you may not have much of an appetite, but it will come roaring back. Many patients worry that they'll be put on a restrictive diet after surgery. Actually, you can eat whatever you want. There's no need to change your diet from before the surgery unless, of course, you were eating like a pig in the first place. If that's the case, take this opportunity to improve your eating habits. Increase your intake of protein with lean meat. Eat more raw fruits and vegetables. Minimize sugars and avoid fats.

· **Get up slowly.** You may feel lightheaded if you get up too quickly from a supine position. *Supine* means lying on your back. Remember to move slowly. Sit at the side of the bed for a few moments, and then get up with some assistance. Have someone help you!

- **Take stairs slowly.** If you must climb stairs, take them one at a time. If you become tired, sit down and rest. Don't keep going until you get so lightheaded that you faint, and risk falling and opening your wounds.

- **Beware of overexcited pets.** If you live with animals, be careful not to allow them to jump or climb on you while the incisions are healing.

- **Don't examine your surgery.** You will feel the urge to look at your surgery. I recommend that you don't for a day or two. Immediately postop there will be some bruising, swelling, and numbness, and for those not accustomed to seeing these postoperative sequelae, the experience can be disheartening. This is further exaggerated by the effects of an anesthesia and pain medication on your emotional state, so don't do it. You'll make yourself crazy. I mean it: *Don't* do it.

- **Remember that there are drugs in your system.** While the anesthesia is wearing off and you're taking pain medication, you are under the influence of drugs. I shouldn't have to tell you what *not* to do while under the influence, but I will anyway.

- **Don't operate heavy machinery.** That means that you can't drive cars or fly airplanes. Don't even skateboard.

- **Don't drink alcohol.** You have a narcotic on board for pain control, so don't complicate it with a depressant. In fact, you should ideally avoid alcohol for at least six weeks following the operation. I know, I know, fat chance, but try it anyway. And yes, beer and wine are alcohol.

What to Expect: Day Three through Day Twenty-one

You should be starting to feel a bit more human by this point. In fact, by the end of the first week, most of your pain should be gone and your bruises should be fading. It's great that you're feeling better, but you still have a way to go before you are your new, improved self. Take it easy. Don't go to the beach club, the disco, church, or wherever it is that you were planning to go to show off your new contours. Don't do anything you don't have to do, or you risk injuring yourself and jeopardizing your results.

Here's how things should go during this crucial recovery period.

- *The follow-up appointment.* Your follow-up appointments with your surgeon should be scheduled for the first postoperative day and a few days after the surgery. Don't worry about not being able to go; you will be feeling better and eager to be up and around. Most of your complaining will have stopped by this time, which your doctor will appreciate.
- *Stay home.* I know you're getting cabin fever, but don't leave your house unless it's necessary. Remember, you just had surgery and you're still recuperating. If you decide to venture out, cover your operative areas with clothing or sunblock. Let someone else drive.
- *Monitor your temperature.* Early in the postoperative period, an increased temperature may indicate that you are not expanding your lungs by taking deep breaths. By days three through five, though, it may be indicative of infection. If your temperature is greater than 101° Fahrenheit, and *only* if it is greater than 101°, call the doctor. He will need to check the incision lines for signs of infection.

· ***Don't overdo it with the pain medication.*** Watch the amount of pain medication that you take. It's not that you can get hooked—that's ludicrous. The problem is constipation. Narcotics slow down your bowels. If you think the surgery was painful, wait until you experience the pleasure of someone manually disimpacting your bowels. Go easy on the pain meds, but there is no need to suffer. Your prescription may run out after a few days, but it is appropriate in many instances to receive a refill.

· ***Expect swelling.*** You will notice an increase in the amount of swelling around the operative site. This is normal and reached its peak at about one week postoperatively.

· ***Expect to urinate frequently.*** After a week, you may find that you have to urinate more than usual. That's your body getting rid of excess fluid as the swelling subsides.

· ***Bandages can be removed.*** After the first week, there is no need to have bandages anymore. In fact, you should remove them.

· ***Wash your wound.*** Wash the wound three times a day with soap and water and apply Bacitracin or Neosporin ointment to the incision line. The ointment is used for one purpose: to keep the crusting from drying so that at the next wash, the wound is easier to clean. I'm not concerned with the antibiotic in the ointment. It probably doesn't do anything anyway. Don't use hydrogen peroxide on the incision. Peroxide does kill bacteria, but it will also kill fibroblasts. Fibroblasts are the cells that make scars. Using peroxide will actually slow down healing, and we don't want that, do we?

· ***Wash the rest of your body.*** Yes, you can take a shower even though the sutures are still in.

· ***Pick your scab.*** I know your grandmother used to tell you not to pick a scab, but she was 100 percent wrong. Keep the incision line perfectly clean. The crusting and scabbing can lead to increased inflammation and separation of the wound edges. This results in increased deposition of collagen and therefore more scarring. So keep it clean.

- **Have your sutures removed.** After five to seven days, the wound is healed enough to hold together on its own. Removing the sutures at this time can help avoid railroad track–type scars—the kind with evenly spaced dots on either side of the wound. Railroad track scars are caused by leaving the sutures in too long. So get them out at the appropriate time suggested by the doctor.

Three Weeks After Surgery

After three weeks, your wounds should be about 80 percent healed and you'll feel 100 percent better. Your incision line may now feel bumpy. That's normal. Your body is producing collagen to make the final scar. In time, this bumpiness will go away.

Now you are ready to resume your routine and start showing off the new you. Here's some advice for getting back to your normal life.

- **Return to work.** Many people return to work after three weeks. Just be careful not to overdo it.
- **Exercise.** Now is the time to resume or start an exercise program. Again, go slowly. It may take a while to get back to the fitness level you were at before surgery, but by six weeks you should be back to normal. Ideally, I'd like you to aim to be a bit more active than you were before surgery. If you were not exercising, now is the time to begin. Physical activity will make your body strong and keep it young, so get off the couch. Join a gym. Do something.

· ***It's OK to resume intimacy.*** Everyone asks about resuming sex with their partner. I suggest waiting until three weeks postop, but the rule of thumb is to go slowly and gently until you are completely comfortable.

· ***Be patient with the healing process.*** You feel better, but you're not completely healed and you haven't seen the final results of your surgery. Much of your bruising and swelling have abated, but not all of it. You may still be disappointed in your appearance. Again, that's normal. Give it time. It can take up to six months to see the final result.

Three Months After Surgery

You'll have another follow-up appointment with your surgeon at about three months after your surgery. He or she will take "after" photographs, and you'll review them together with the "before" pictures. You'll be amazed and thrilled at the change.

One Year After Surgery

At some point around eight to twelve months postop, everything you went through—preparing for the surgery, the surgery itself, and the recovery process—will all fade into a hazy memory. Your scars will have flattened and faded. You will be completely comfortable and at home with the new you. You will be glad you did it. Your new look will be yours.

5

Scarring and Wound Healing

SCARS ARE ONE OF the primary concerns of all women of color considering a surgical procedure. That's because dark skin (i.e., skin with increased melanin) is more prone to thick, unsightly scars than light skin. After all, what's the point of having cosmetic surgery in order to feel better about your appearance if you wind up with a disfiguring scar?

Scarring—how wounds heal—is a complicated process that has many variables. It's difficult to predict who will develop prominent scars and who won't. But there are ways to diminish thick scars, should they occur.

We'll use the case history of one of my favorite young patients to explore the problem of scarring and what can be done about it.

Gwendolyn's Story

When I met Gwendolyn, I had been in practice only six months. I walked into the examination room one day to find an attractive black woman in her early forties sitting in one chair. In another chair sat her eleven-year-old daughter. The child didn't even look up as I entered the room.

"Hi, I'm Dr. Adams," I said.

A sigh of relief came across the woman's face with that announcement. I suppose it was at the realization that I'm black. Sometimes patients are shocked rather than relieved by my appearance. I'm used to both reactions by now. I guess America isn't quite ready for me yet.

"Who's Gwendolyn?" I asked. The woman pointed to the young girl, who hardly flinched on hearing her name. She continued reading, trying desperately to ignore me.

"Well, Gwendolyn," I said. "Let's get you to take a seat over there." I pointed to the examination chair. "What brings you to the office today?"

Gwendolyn, though quiet and shy, was a pleasant eleven-year-old black girl. She was larger than her age would indicate, though it certainly could not be said she was overweight. She was athletic, and much more developed physically than one would expect of an eleven-year-old.

Her face was full and round, with large full lips. Her hair was in long flowing braids with beads at the end. Her eyes, though large and sparkling, avoided contact with mine.

Her voice was soft and high-pitched, and it was this that most clearly betrayed her age. I felt drawn to her immediately.

She had come for evaluation of what her mother described as keloid scars on her face. Keloids are thick, mushrooming scars that can be very disfiguring.

Gwendolyn had been in a motor vehicle accident three months earlier and had sustained multiple facial lacerations. The accident occurred while she was on the school bus. At the time of the accident she was treated by an emergency room physician. Her mother was bringing her to me now because she had become concerned about the scars.

Gwendolyn was self-conscious about the way she looked. Her preoccupation had changed her personality. She was more introverted and participating less in school activities. Her mother was understandably worried.

When I examined Gwendolyn, I saw that she had three significant scars. One near her left ear was over two inches long; there was an inch-and-a-half-long scar on her forehead; and a thick two-inch scar on her lower face made her chin and neck look uneven and tilted to the right. However, they were hypertrophic scars, not keloids.

I explained to Gwendolyn and her mother that the scars were not the dreaded keloids. "That's good news," I said, "because unlike keloids, hypertrophic scars eventually begin to get smaller."

Both Gwendolyn and her mother gave me their full attention. Gwendolyn put down her book and began to make eye contact with me.

"How can you tell the difference between hypertrophic scars and keloids?" asked Gwendolyn's mother. It was a good question. Many people confuse the two, though they are significantly different. Gwendolyn was listening intently, eager for more information, so I spelled out the differences.

I advised them to think of scarring as occurring on a continuum. At one end is a perfect, fine-line scar, while on other end is the thick, mushrooming keloid scar. Hypertropic scars, like the ones on Gwendolyn's face, are somewhere in the middle.

Types of Scars

- *Fine-line scars.* Ideally, healthy, mature scar tissue will form a thin line over the original incision, tightly joining the two sides of the wound together. It may be slightly raised, but should be close to the color of the surrounding skin.
- *Hypertrophic scars.* These are wide, flat scars that look thin and stretched. They can be thick like keloids, but they have less collagen and their boundaries are within the original wound. As they mature, they tend to diminish in size. They occur most often in people with dark skin.
- *Keloid scars.* Keloids are scars that can grow to look like mushrooms or cauliflower. They are actually benign tumors that grow until they incorporate skin that was not part of the initial wound. In a keloid, collagen, which is the material that makes up the scar, overgrows and extends out to invade

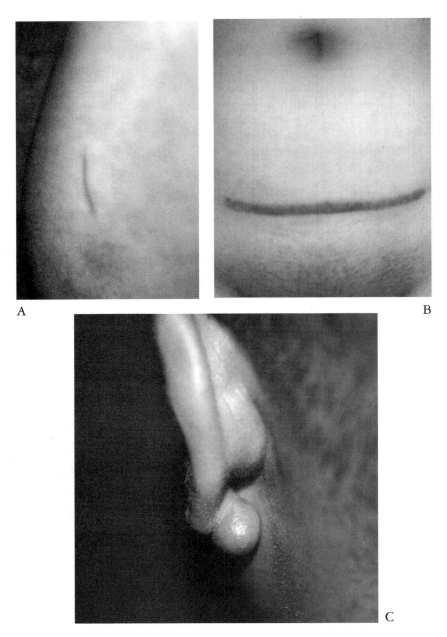

A

B

C

Figure 4: Scarring is the result of two processes: a mechanical process, which is controlled by the surgeon, and a biological process, which is wound healing.
A. Fine-line scar; B. Hypertrophic scar; C. Keloid.

the surrounding tissue. This kind of scarring occurs most often in young, dark-skinned patients. The scars usually continue to grow without signs of spontaneous regression; that is, they don't get smaller with time.

"Doctor, if Gwendolyn has hypertrophic scars that are going to diminish, when will that happen?" asked the mother. Gwendolyn nodded vigorously, seconding the question.

"It's important to understand that scars take a very long time to reach their final form—sometimes as long as a year and a half," I answered. "Would you like me to explain what your body does to fix itself after you get a cut?" I asked Gwendolyn. She nodded shyly, so I began to elaborate on the scarring process.

How Scars Are Formed

The first thing to understand is that scars are the result of two actions:

- **Wound closure:** This is a mechanical process controlled by the surgeon through his gentleness to the tissue and how much tension is on the final wound.
- **Healing:** This is a biological process, and everyone heals differently. Some people, particularly the young and those with dark skin, are prone to hypertrophic or even keloid scars. The formation of a keloid scar is not dependent on the skill of the surgeon. It is the result of an aberration in the biological aspects of wound healing. Normally, injury causes a local response in the wounded tissue. That response, which is what we call "wound healing," occurs in three phases.
- **The inflammatory phase.** The first stage is the formation of *granulation tissue.* Granulation tissue is the pink tissue that

forms first in a wound. In this phase, small blood vessels dilate and there is an increase in capillary permeability. *Permeability* is the passage of liquids back and forth across the vessel wall. Permeability is the process that results in swelling. White blood cells migrate into the wound to clean it. They, in turn, are followed by fibroblasts, which are the cells that make the scar material. Fibroblasts fuse the intercellular matrix into granulation tissue, the glue that holds the two sides of a wound together. This occurs during the first five days after an injury.

· *The fibroplasia stage phase.* In the second stage of wound healing, the granulation tissue is transformed into normal young connective tissue. During this time, the wound changes from a fine-line scar to a thick red one. This takes place as the fibroblasts form collagen to close the wound. This period occurs approximately from day five to day twenty-one. By the end of this phase, the wound should be about 80 percent healed. At this point you should be able to resume your normal activities.

· *The maturation phase.* In the last phase of healing, the tissue evolves into a mature scar. The final form of the tissue depends on the type of stresses applied to the wound, so the look and feel of the scar depends upon the function of the tissue that is injured. For example, scar tissue on your thumb, which you move and use constantly, will be different than scar tissue on your scalp, which does not need to have the same flexibility and mobility. The tissue keeps growing and changing until it reaches the necessary tensile strength—that is, it can resist the forces trying to pull the wound apart. When the scar tissue is as strong as the undamaged tissue surrounding it, the healing process is complete. This phase can take up to a year and a half.

That's the healing process when it works correctly. Sometimes things don't happen quite so neatly. Normal wound healing can be affected by a number of factors, both internal and external. These include things like infection, tension or pressure on the wound, blood clotting, nutrition, and hormonal influence.

Are You at Risk for Developing Keloids?

None of these factors seem to specifically cause keloids. The development of keloid scars is unpredictable and occurs under apparently normal healing conditions. In fact, in phase one, the inflammatory phase, the wound heals as it should. Yet, instead of moving into the fibroplasia phase, the granulation tissue continues to grow and involve the surrounding skin. The collagen in the scar keeps accumulating instead of breaking down and becoming refined as it does in hypertrophic and fine-line scars.

At this point Gwendolyn's mother interrupted with a question: "But I was thinking about a tummy tuck myself. How can I tell if I'm going to have keloids?"

I explained that, unfortunately, there is no existing biological test to predict who will form a keloid and who will not. What causes keloid formation is still unknown. There are, however, indicators that make it possible to tell if you have a higher than normal risk of developing them.

- **Age.** People between ages ten and thirty are most likely to form keloids.
- **Sex.** Women are more likely than men to develop keloids.
- **Skin color.** Dark-skinned people experience keloids more often than fair-skinned people.

· **Family history.** If a relative had keloids, you are more likely to develop them than someone without any family history of keloids.

Solutions to Scarring

I could tell I was slowly earning their trust. Gwendolyn had become more attentive and her face was animated. I had given them information about what was happening to Gwendolyn so that they could understand their options and make decisions concerning her future therapy.

Finally, Gwendolyn herself spoke up. "Dr. Adams, what can we do about *my* scars?"

I leaned toward her and made eye contact. I wanted to make certain she understood everything. But I also wanted her to believe in me because I wanted to help her. Overcoming the psychological hurdle of having facial scars is never easy, especially at such a tender age.

"There are two ways to approach the problem of scarring," I told her. "We can either do more surgery to try to get them under control, or we can try different types of nonsurgical management. The nonsurgical approach means no more cutting, which most people prefer."

I went on to explain the options in more detail.

Nonsurgical Scar Management Options

· ***Corticosteroids.*** This medication is injected into the scar tissue. It is theoretically designed to be used during the first phase of wound healing—the inflammatory phase—to decrease the amount of granulation tissue and other substances that result in the final scar. Steroids can also be used in the later stages of healing; they decrease the size of the scar by decreasing the amount of scar material in the wound.

- **Pressure garments.** The application of Ace wraps or silicone gel pads helps flatten out the scar. This therapy works best during the maturation phase. The silicone pads work because of a physical-chemical reaction. According to one theory, the negative charges of the silicone cause the scar to align so that it is flat. Another theory is that the gel sheet facilitates scar hydration and occlusion.
- **X rays.** The scar tissue is irradiated with X rays. Again, this therapy is designed to be used during the inflammatory phase to reduce the production of granulation tissue.
- **Lasers.** Laser treatments have gotten a lot of press lately, but they are not always a good option, especially for people of color. Many different types of lasers have been tested in the treatment of scars. The first was the CO_2 laser. Lasers are gentle to tissue and display certain anti-inflammatory properties. There were high hopes that this would be ideal for suppressing keloid formation. However, in practice, lasers were not found to suppress the growth or the recurrence of keloids. The argon and Nd: YAG lasers have also been tried, but not specifically in women of color because of possible thermal injury. Lasers work by the wavelength of light they produce, which generates heat to selectively destroy structures that absorb the light. The melanin in the skin of people of color also absorbs the light, and therefore the heat. This makes the destruction of tissue and structures less selective. This is the reason laser therapy is not a good option for people of color. The good news is that a number of companies are developing machines that use wider wavelengths of light, and these may prove beneficial for people of color in the future.
- **Colchicine.** This alkaloid medication is normally used for gout, but it has been known to disrupt collagen synthesis and also stimulate its breakdown. Though it sounds promising,

so far it has been used on scars with minimal success. Colchicine functions to decrease wound contraction, decrease the number of inflammatory cells in the wound, and control the production of granulation tissue. To be effective at all, it would have to be administered early in phase one.

· *Antihistamines.* These drugs have been used in the treatment of hypertrophic scars, but again without much success. Antihistamines, along with other drugs, delay wound healing and are immunosuppressive. To be effective, they would have to work early in phase one of the healing process.

· *Zinc.* Zinc influences wound healing by reducing free radical activity, improving cell mitosis and proliferation, strengthening collagen cross-bonding, and inhibiting bacterial growth. Valuable sources of zinc include red meats, nuts, and cereals. Care must be taken in using zinc supplements, though, because these can cause abdominal pain and lower serum levels of copper, and inhibit the effectiveness of some antibiotics, including tetracycline.

· *Vitamin E.* Vitamin E gained a lot of attention when it was shown to be beneficial in lowering the risk of coronary artery disease. However, it should be discontinued prior to surgery. It has been found to impair wound healing and collagen synthesis. However, in scars it may prove beneficial if administered early in phase two.

· *Retin-A.* Vitamin A restores the inflammatory phase of wound healing in those individuals whose wound healing has been impaired by steroids. In addition, Vitamin A favorably influences the immune depression seen in patients as a result of injury, sepsis, or surgery. Its benefits may be in those people who are immune-deficient.

Surgical Scar Management

Because the healing process is so complex and slow, plastic surgeons don't like to surgically revise scars too soon after they form. It is best to wait for the scar to complete the maturation phase before attempting surgical therapy.

Generally, surgery is more useful for keloids than hypertrophic scars. During the procedure, the surgeon cuts away the excess scar tissue and contours the wound to blend with the surrounding tissue.

After surgery, you must use one of the nonsurgical therapies to keep the scar from reforming. Corticosteroids or X ray irradiation are usually the most effective. If you don't follow up with a nonsurgical therapy, there is almost a 100 percent chance that the keloid will reform. Even more frightening, the keloid may come back bigger than it was originally.

Gwendolyn's Treatment

Gwendolyn and her mother looked hopeful. For the first time, they really seemed to believe that something could be done to improve the appearance of her scars.

"In your case," I said finally, "we need to give the scars more time to mature, say six months or so. I know that's easy for me to say because it isn't happening to me. But maturation has to be the first line of business. After that, we can consider injections with a steroid, or surgical revision. Right now I would just give them time."

Reluctantly, Gwendolyn accepted my advice and her mother scheduled a follow-up visit for six months later.

When they returned, Gwendolyn's scars had finished maturing. They were still raised, but the color matched the surrounding skin. Surgery didn't seem necessary, so I opted to inject them with Kenalog 40, a steroid.

I saw her three weeks later, and the therapy was working. The scars were flattening out to approximate the level of the surrounding skin. The color match was perfect. I even imagined that there was less tension from the scar pulling on the surrounding tissue. She was happy with the result and even smiled. I saw her one more time three months after that. I was certain that the desired effect, flattening and thinning of the hypertrophic scars, would have taken place. I just needed to be sure. Your heart goes out when you see this happening to a child, particularly a young girl.

The scars had completely flattened. The color match of the skin was also good. There was, however, some difference in the texture between the scar and the normal skin, but this was to be expected, and frankly, was of little consequence to Gwendolyn since things were going well. There was no reason to schedule another return visit. Gwendolyn's face was hers again.

"Give me a call if you have any questions or problems," I said.

She nodded and went away a very happy young girl.

6

Skin Care

THE FOUNDATION OF ALL beauty is skin care. The skin is the largest organ of the body, and any discussion about beauty and beauty solutions must begin with a discussion of the skin, its functions, and its care.

Skin: The Protective Barrier

Your skin's main function is to protect you. It is a large elastic, waterproof, and self-repairing barrier. It protects the body from mechanical injuries that are the result of physical forces. Mechanical injury can result from stretching, twisting, pressure, or cutting. And it also protects us from our environment, which can be hostile. Bacteria, viruses, toxic chemicals, and the like have difficulty penetrating the skin to infect the organism underneath. We all come into contact with millions of bacteria and microorganisms every day and, contrary to what conventional knowledge would have us believe, very few of us come down with infections. The reality is that your skin is so good at what it does that infections don't usually occur unless you have a cut or some break in the skin. When your skin is well taken care of, it shields the body heroically.

Skin: The Sense Organ

Of course, your skin is clearly more than a protective shield that protects your vital fluids and tissues from injury. It is also a sense organ, one that allows us to interact with our environment. The skin is an instrument of expression that responds to our feelings. It displays our emotions quickly and vividly. Fear, excitement, and embarrassment are displayed as sweating, a change in color (either redness or blueness), or blushing. We also experience our environment through our sense of touch. Our skin conveys hot or cold, wet or dry, soft or hard, and sharp or dull.

Skin: The Excretory Organ

Your skin is also an excretory organ. Toxic chemicals can be eliminated from your body through evaporation, incuding injested substances such as alcohol. The skin is also a heat control organ; sweating is the body's way of cooling down.

Your skin is so reliable and effective that we hardly appreciate it or take notice of it until a problem presents itself. This is a mistake. Given all your skin does for you, taking care of it should be a health and beauty priority. In fact, if you want to stay beautiful, you *must* take good care of your skin. There are a number of things that you can do to protect your skin and to help it perform its functions while maintaining a youthful glow. Perhaps the most important of these is to *establish a beauty regimen that works for you and stick to it.* That regimen should include the three skin care basics:

1. Cleansing
2. Moisturizing
3. Sun protection

We will talk more about this regimen later, including how to personalize it to fit your individual needs.

Believe it or not, physicians themselves are partly to blame for our failure to make skin care an important priority in our lives. Doctors tend to view most skin disorders as nothing more than blemishes—they treat them as nuisances rather than serious problems. This clearly is wrong and, frankly, insensitive. We all need to evaluate our skin, its functions, its diseases, and its deterioration with aging. Particularly, our society must start paying attention to the physical and psychological stresses caused by the deterioration in the appearance of skin.

Children have relatively few skin problems. By the time we reach age sixty-five, most of us will have at least two skin problems that are worthy of medical attention. As our skin ages, it becomes weaker. It sweats less, loses pigment, heals less quickly, and becomes cooler in temperature. It's thinner, looser, dryer, and can get scaly and rough.

Suzanne's Sorrow

When Suzanne showed up in my office, she was concerned that her skin was experiencing many of the adverse effects of aging listed above. Her main anxiety, however, was that the skin on her cheeks had become blotchy and there was an accumulation of dark freckles on her face and neck. This fifty-four-year-old black woman, a schoolteacher, was literally in tears during our first meeting. She had seen at least fifteen doctors in Beverly Hills and no one would treat her problems. Frankly, she had been ignored because many of those physicians feared that treatment would result in a keloid, pigmentary changes, or simply horrible scarring. Some of the physicians had even tried to discourage her with the old adage that it's what's inside that counts, as if appearances in this case didn't matter. Suzanne, however, knew all too well that while individuals with heart disease or cancer receive empathy and understanding, those with skin disorders can be rejected and compromised in all interpersonal relationships.

Physically, Suzanne was healthy. But psychologically, she was a mess. I felt for her because I knew she was in pain. There was no escaping the spots she saw on her face in the mirror every morning. She just didn't feel good about herself. Her problem had become so important in her life that it had literally changed her personality. She had gone from being a very social person who had a great many friends to being isolated and lonely. She was single now and had even stopped dating because she had become too self-conscious. As she told me how she felt, I didn't interrupt. I didn't try to explain away what she was feeling. I just let her cry. I wanted her to know that I was listening.

Many women of color like Suzanne have been miseducated about skin care and aging. Most scientific studies about aging skin have focused on Caucasian skin, with reference made to people of color only when it helps to clarify an issue concerning white skin. This has led to erroneous conclusions about what is going on in the skin of people of color. There are a number of basic differences between black and white skin, the most obvious being color.

In all skin types there are four different kinds of cells. The predominant type is the keratinocyte cell, which is the main structural component of skin. Langerhans and Merkel cells defend against bacteria and other microorganisms. The fourth type is the malanocyte, which is the cell that produces pigment. Interestingly, there is no difference in the number of melanocyte cells between black and white skin. The differences in skin color are the result of how much pigment is produced, and how and where it is stored in the keratinocyte. Pigment is produced in the melanocyte and packaged in granules called *melanosomes.* The melanosomes are then transferred to the keratinocyte. In whites, the melanosomes are smaller and dispersed in groups inside the keratinocyte. In blacks, the melanosomes are larger and dispersed individually inside keratinocytes.

While the outer layer of skin—called the *stratum corneum*—is of equal thickness in blacks and whites, blacks have an increased number of cell layers and more lipids (fats) in the skin. Furthermore, sunlight demonstrates an increased phototransmission in whites, but there is an increased photoprotection in blacks. That is, the melanin in black skin serves to prevent the ultraviolet radiation from penetrating the skin and causing damage. This is precisely what has posed the greatest problems in skin care for women of color. While it is true that the melanin in dark skin makes it somewhat more photoprotective than white skin, it does not make it a coat of armor.

When physicians speak of the skin's aging process, we are really talking about two different but related processes. We define skin aging as *intrinsic* or *extrinsic*.

- *Intrinsic, chronologic aging* refers to aging as a result of time. How you age intrinsically has a lot to do with your family background and genetic makeup. Your skin is most likely going to age along the lines of your mother or grandmother. Intrinsically aged skin is thinner and more transparent than young skin, which often makes blood vessels become visible under the skin's surface. Older skin loses its elasticity, causing it to sag and wrinkle. The dermis, which is the deeper layer of skin, is also thinner and therefore doesn't have the same ability to perform its barrier function, making it harder to clear chemical substances, regulate temperature, and heal properly.
- *Extrinsic aging,* now often referred to as *photo-aging* because it is related to sun exposure, is the supposition of photo-damage on the aging process. Extrinsic aging occurs as a result of injury from environmental influences, including ultraviolet radiation, smoking, wind, and exposure to chemicals. Photo-aged skin is characterized by an exaggeration of the changes seen in intrinsic aging, as well as by the addi-

tional damage caused by exposure to ultraviolet rays, or sunlight. The sun is the major cause of fine lines, dark spots, and
skin cancers.

In white skin, extrinsic damage is usually manifested in a ruddy,
coarse complexion, pebbly, irregular pigmentation, the presence of
fine blood vessels, and fine and coarse skin wrinkles. Sun exposure
can also cause the development of basal and squamous cell carcino-
mas, the skin cancers, as well as melanomas in light skin.

In women of color the effects of extrinsic damage are often
less obvious. The onset of wrinkling may be delayed for decades.
Still, the hyperpigmentation and dark spots that trouble many
women of color *do represent sun damage.* These dark spots are the result, or rather the response, of melanocytes to injury by the sun.
There are two common cutaneous conditions that affect women of
color as a result of aging and sun damage: *dermatosis papulosa nigra*
and *melasma.*

· **Dermatosis Papulosa Nigra (DPN)** affects more than
half of African-American adults, though women have a
higher incidence than men. DPN is characterized by dark
brown to black spots that resemble freckles, called *papules.*
Usually they begin to appear on the skin when you're in your
twenties or thirties. They are found most commonly on the
cheeks, though it is also possible to have them on your neck,
arms, and trunk. With time, they increase in size, number,
and location, some reaching 2 centimeters in diameter. They
continue to grow in size and number until you are sixty or
seventy years old. After this time, new ones seldom appear.
· **Melasma** is a mottled discoloration of the sun-exposed areas of the face. Sometimes the discoloration is symmetric.
The pigmentation changes, either hyperpigmentation (dark

spots) or hypopigmentation (lightened areas), are most prominent on the cheeks, forehead, upper lip, chin, and nose. Sometimes the dark patches or hyperpigmentation occur around the eyes. It is most often seen in light-skinned African-American women and Latinas. The cause is unknown, but it may be associated with pregnancy or oral estrogen-containing contraceptives (although many women who have neither been pregnant nor take birth control pills may be affected). It is possible that this condition is hereditary in nature, but there is no doubt that sun exposure complicates the problem and contributes to its worsening with age.

There is another rare condition called *actinic keratosis* that can cause premalignant warty lesions on the skin. This condition, like the others, is accentuated by sun exposure.

After Suzanne finished her story and collected herself, she asked, "These ugly dark spots on my face, what do you think they are? I've tried everything and none of the doctors I've seen seem to be able to do anything about them."

I wished to help her by giving her the information she wanted to hear, but I had to be honest: I told her I wasn't sure what was causing her problem and I wasn't sure that I had a solution.

Suzanne was at the end of her rope. "Well, what *do* you know?" she demanded.

I began by explaining what was happening to her skin. Basically, the melanocyte, the cell in her skin that makes pigment, was overactive. Melanocytes are always more active in dark-skinned people than in those with light skin. It is precisely this activity, if you will, that leads to disturbances of pigmentation when the cells are injured.

Dark skin is a defense against the harmful effects of the sun, but there's more to it than that. The melanocyte is also involved in performing other important functions. It responds to threats of injury, be they from the outside or from inside the body. Think of it this way: Hyperpigmentation may be a sign that the pigment is performing its duty to help maintain homeostasis. Homeostasis is the ability of the body to maintain a balance of various functions in spite of constantly being challenged by outside forces like heat and cold, bacteria or viruses, or inside forces like lack of nutrition.

Melanocytes also help combat free radicals. Everyone's heard of free radicals, but what exactly are they? Free radical production may be the final common denominator in producing substances that cause injury to cells. They are actually intermediates in the reaction. For example, if you put hydrogen and oxygen together, you can make water, but first the electrons have to change orbits as they begin to share the electron to form the finished product. Just before water is formed, these free electrons are floating around; they are what's known as free radicals. We know that vitamins or antioxidants help rid the body of free radicals. And so does melanin. Melanin is found in the cytoplasm, or body, of keratinocytes. It assists in scavenging free radicals. It removes them from the cell, and that helps to stop cell injury. This may be the reason black people have fewer skin cancers.

"So when I see these dark spots on people," I concluded, "I have to ask, what threats of injury or what noxious stimuli is their skin responding to?"

Suzanne gave me an indignant stare that I'd never seen before. She was actually disgusted. Finally, she spoke up. "So what?" she asked.

"What do you mean, so what?" I responded.

"I mean, so what? You go on and on about melanocytes this and hyperpigmentation that. A lot of big words, but they don't mean a thing for me. I still have to deal psychologically day in and day out with the fact that I have these dark patches on my face and around my eyes. I don't feel good about myself. It stops me from being the outgoing person I am. I'm single and I don't meet men because I'm too self-conscious, and so I say so what? I want to know what I can do to help me."

"Wait a minute," I said to Suzanne. "Slow down. It's not about so what, it's about understanding the cause. The cause gives you an idea of what you need to do to correct it. We need to understand the functions of the melanocyte and melanin in order to discover where things went wrong and what you and I can do to solve *your* problem."

The first step, I told her, was to take a look at some of the possible causes of hyperpigmentation. The list of potential causes is enormous, and it is impossible to catalog them all, but it can be helpful to go through the most likely explanations. If one of these factors was causing her dark patches, we could cure her problem merely by discontinuing it. Here are some of the causes we considered:

- **Endocrine factors,** including a variety of hormones such as melanocyte-stimulating hormone, estrogens, testosterone, and glucocorticoids.
- **Chemical and pharmacologic agents,** such as the fatty acids (arachidonic acid or limoleic acid).
- **Mechanical injury and skin trauma,** such as cuts, bruises, or burns.
- **Inflammatory diseases,** such as acne and dermatitis.
- **Cancer drugs,** including Bleomycin, 5-fluorouracil, methotrexate, and Adriamycin.
- **Tetracycline drugs,** used in the treatment of minor infections, including urinary tract infections and acne.
- **Anti-malarial drugs,** like Puromethamine.
- **Metals,** including iron, lead, mercury, silver, and arsenic. Patients may be exposed to these metals either through their vocation, or they can be injected (i.e., increased iron intake leading to hemochromatosis).

- **Nitrous compounds,** like aniline dye, which is prepared from benzene and serves as the basis of many brilliant dyes and in the manufacture of plastics.
- **Hormones.** This includes hormones your own body produces: Adrenocorticotrophic hormone, ACTH, and melanin-stimulating hormone, MSH, can cause a dark brown color of the skin. Estrogen can also cause a brownish color of skin folds and hyperpigmentation around the nipple areolar complex.
- **Birth control pills.** Birth control pills mimic pregnancy, and you can tell if a woman has had children just by looking at her stomach and seeing that dark line that goes down the center. Well, that dark line is the linea alba, which has darkened in response to the hormones of pregnancy.

Suzanne's past medical history didn't give many clues. She had no history of hormonal or endocrine disease; there was no contact with any chemical or pharmacological agents that would trigger an inflammatory response; nor had she experienced any mechanical injury or trauma. However, she had taken birth control pills in the past and had two children, both grown, ages thirty-one and twenty-eight. She'd had a hysterectomy three years earlier, and at the present time was experiencing symptoms of menopause including hot flashes and sweating.

The Pill and the pregnancies could explain some of her pigmentation problems, but the time frame of the lesions did not coincide.

Her family history, although positive for diabetes and high blood pressure, gave no clue as to the reason for the dark spots.

We couldn't pinpoint the cause of Suzanne's hyperpigmentation by going through this list, so we moved on to discussing what we could—and could not—do about the problem. I told her the next step was to determine whether the melanin was deposited in the *dermis* or the *epidermis* of her skin. The epidermis is the outer layer of skin. There are no blood vessels in the epidermis. The dermis is the active layer of skin, which has blood vessels and nerves coursing through it. We would need to biopsy the skin in order to locate the level of the pigment. This is important because the two types of deposits represent very different situations.

If the melanin is deposited in the dermis, you've got a problem, I told her. We have no medications that are able to destroy melanin located at this level. Melanin deposited in the keratinocytes, however, is a different story. The keratinocytes start in the deep layers of the skin, and they migrate to the surface, carrying melanin with them as they age. Eventually, the melanin is lost with dead skin cells.

If the pigment is in the epidermis, the problem can be addressed by reducing the melanocyte's production of melanin. This can be done with topical medications that you rub into your skin. This treatment takes a long time; realistically, it can take a year or more. Hydroquinone, a lightening cream, applied two or three times a day, will resolve the problem somewhat, though you may have to use it forever. If that doesn't work, a topical steroid can be added to your regimen. Excellent results have been demonstrated with this combination of Hydroquinone and steroids. Other things that we can consider are chemical peels, particularly with trichloracetic acid, or TCA.

I stressed that along with what we would try to do to correct the problem, Suzanne needed to practice prevention. That is, she had to avoid the sun. *The sun is clearly the major cause of this kind of damage* and subsequent hyperpigmentation of the skin. I suggested that she begin using a sunscreen and a moisturizer with antioxidants while we waited for the results of her biopsy.

Protecting the Skin

I urge all my patients to practice a healthy skin care regimen. I can't overstress how important this is. Your skin is assaulted by so many forces—sun, gravity, disease—that it needs all the help it can get.

As we discussed, there are two basic processes that cause the characteristic changes that we see in the skin with aging. One is caused by age itself, the other by sun damage. In addition to these intrinsic and extrinsic signs of aging, which all people experience, there are a number of skin problems associated with aging that are more prominent in blacks than whites.

- *Increased pigment lability,* resulting in frequent hyper- and hypopigmentation. The skin for the most part is composed of four cell types: keratinocytes (90 percent), Langerhans and Merkel cells (5 percent), and pigment cells (5 percent). The pigment cells were thought to be relatively passive cells. Ultraviolet light was well known to increase the activity of these cells, resulting in tanning; however, it is now known that the activity and proliferation of melanocytes can be either stimulated or inhibited by a wide variety of factors, including injury and a variety of hormones.
- *Follicular responses and follicular diseases* (blackheads, ingrown hairs). Because of the relative coarseness of the hair in people of color, disturbances, either as a result of injury or bacteria, can occur at the level of the hair follicle. This repeated injury as a result of inflammation can lead to the formation of cysts, abscesses, blackheads and whiteheads, and ingrown hairs.
- *Fibroplastic and granulomatous changes* (*dermatosus papulosa nigra*). If the injuries to the skin become chronic, the

constant inflammation can lead to excessive scarring and pigmented growths that may resemble freckles at first, but with time continue to grow forming dark skin tags. Skin tags are small growths or elevations of the skin. They are benign, not cancerous, and do not contain pus.

What all this means is that you must take good care of your skin to keep it healthy and avoid these conditions. In response to hundreds of patients like Suzanne, I developed a basic skin care regimen to help them avoid future skin problems. It is designed to be used throughout your lifetime, and it takes into account the changes in your skin's needs as it ages.

The results of Suzanne's biopsy demonstrated that the increased melanin pigment was located in both the dermis and the epidermis. While the finding of epidermal location was good news, the dermal location was not. Nevertheless, I felt that if we could address the epidermal melanin, she would have considerable improvement.

Four percent hydroquinone, along with corticosteroid, was applied to the lesions three times a day for approximately eight months, with fantastic results.

Suzanne was pleased, and so was I.

Skin Care Basics

The period up to puberty is the preventive phase of skin care, and a few smart things done regularly can go far to avoid problems in the future. By age thirty or forty, we all have some dark spots or freckles or fine lines, and we wonder how this happened and what can we do. It's important to understand that these signs of aging are all a result of over thirty years of sun exposure, and while we cannot completely avoid the sun, there are some things that we can do to help decrease its effect.

There are three skin care basics that you should practice throughout your life, starting in childhood. They are *cleansing, moisturizing,* and *protecting.*

CLEANSING

As with most things, there is a right way and a wrong way to wash your face. You don't want to irritate your skin when you cleanse it. Always use a non-soap cleanser that is pH balanced, to get rid of any impurities without stripping the skin of its delicate acid mantle. I recommend that you use your fingers rather than an abrasive cloth. As we discussed earlier, the melanocytes, which respond to injury and irritation, are contributing factors in the blotchiness of the face that is the result of areas of either hyper- or hypopigmentation. Use slightly warm water and massage the cleanser into a lather using your fingertips. Avoid scrubbing your face too hard, as this can injure the melanocytes. Rinse gently with lukewarm water, and pat your face dry.

Here are a few cleansers I recommend:

- Rudalgo's Solution Facial Cleanser
- Rudalgo's Solution Non-soap Cleansing Bar
- Dove Cleansing Bar
- Oil of Olay Cleansing Bar
- Avon Clear Skin

MOISTURIZING AND PROTECTING

Your moisturizer should be a lightweight, greaseless, emollient formula that provides wide-spectrum sun protection against ultraviolet damage. Ideally, this formula should also contain antioxidants, including vitamins A, C, and E, since it is known that ultraviolet light causes oxidative damage in skin and inhibits cutaneous defense systems.

Here are a few moisturizers with sunscreen that I recommend:

- Rudalgo's Solution Facial Moisturizer SPF 30
- Rudalgo's Solution Body Moisturizer SPF 30
- Swiss Formula Body Lotion with Vitamin E
- Avon's Renew Moisturizer

Prepuberty

The period before puberty is the time to develop good skin care habits. A few preventive measures now will pay off later in life. At this age, you just need to cover the basics: Cleanse, moisturize, and protect.

Puberty

Most teens have some trouble with skin blemishes. The onset of puberty, with its attendant increase in hormones, particularly androgens, causes an increase in the size and activity of the glands in the face that secrete oils for lubricating the skin and hair. This, along with sebum, bacteria, and inflammation leads to the formation of blackheads, whiteheads, superficial cysts and pustules, and the condition known as acne. When the cysts rupture, bacteria are released into the tissues, causing an inflammatory reaction that heals with scarring. Over a period of time, the scarring can become very prominent, particularly on the cheeks.

Because of the complex pathogenesis of acne and the fact that it is universal, prevention may not be feasible. Diet appears to have little or no effect. Let's just say that if you have acne, avoid applying cosmetics that contain oils which can block the pores. If the acne is pustular, your doctor can treat it with a four-week regimen of tetracycline. Your physician may also add Retin-A to your routine. This is a topical solution, available by prescription, that makes structural improvements in the skin, including normalization of the epidermis, deposition of new collagen, and new blood vessel formation.

During puberty it is important to continue cleansing with a non-soap pH-balanced cleanser. You may also want to consider occasionally having your skin cleansed by a dermatologist or cosmetician. At this time, a Schamberg loop extractor should be used once or twice a week to clean the pores of any impacted sebum. The Schamberg loop is simply a metal instrument that makes it easier to extrude sebum from the pores. It works better than two fingers. It is also important to use a moisturizer with sunscreen and antioxidants.

Postpuberty

After puberty, skin problems are more common and may require specific treatment. Again, the majority of these problems are related to sun exposure. An effective sunscreen is the key to minimizing brown spots, avoiding fine wrinkles, and starting on the road to improving these kinds of lesions. There are treatments available designed to rejuvenate the skin and address specific problems. However, you should not abandon the good habits that you've developed over the years.

Continue cleaning your face with a non-soap, pH-balanced cleanser and follow with a moisturizer containing sunscreen and antioxidants. You may also need to consider adding some of the following topical therapies:

- **Deep pore cleansing,** such as professional facials.
- **Retin-A.** This is more than an acne medication. When doctors observed that patients with acne develop smoother skin after using Retin-A, it began to be used in the treatment of photo-damaged skin.
- **Alpha and beta hydroxy acid.** These acids, which are made from fruit juices, serve very well in the rejuvena-

tion of the skin by removing superficial dark spots and fine wrinkles. As skin ages, the skin cells move from the deeper layers where the skin is young to the outer layers where the skin is relatively older. These weak acids expose the younger skin by gently removing the older outer layers. An added benefit to the use of alpha and beta hydroxy acids is that they are somewhat sun-protective.

- **Hydroquinone** is the active ingredient in bleaching creams. Hydroquinone blocks the activity of the enzyme tyrosinase, which is important in helping the melanocyte to produce melanin. In a sense, hydroquinone decreases melanin production, thus lightening the skin. It can also be used along with corticosteroids.
- **Kojic acid.** This compound is produced by fungi. It inhibits the formation of melanin by interfering with the uptake of oxygen required to produce the pigment. Kojic acid is supplied as a gel that is massaged into the affected areas two or three times per day. Treatment lasts two to three months.

For more serious skin problems, one or more of the following surgical therapies may be advisable:

- **Chemical peels.** These procedures utilize acids that are stronger than the alpha-hydroxy acids. The most commonly used include trichloracetic acid (TCA) and phenol. Because they are stronger, they burn deeper, removing more layers of skin cells. Thus, care must be taken in their use because burning too deeply can result in scarring.
- **Dermabrasion** involves sanding to remove the superficial layer of cells. It is indicated in acne scarring be-

cause it can help to smooth the cheeks and face. Again, care must be taken not to sand too deeply for fear of creating more scars.

· **Botox.** Botox is short for botulism toxin. This substance is known to paralyze muscles for up to two to three months. The facial wrinkles in the forehead, around the eyes, and at the root of the nose are due to muscle contraction. By injecting Botox directly into the muscle, one can paralyze the muscle and thereby eliminate the wrinkle. The amount of Botox used is nontoxic.

· **Laser Therapy.** This procedure is not usually recommended for women of color. It is important to understand that laser therapy is based on heat; the laser uses light to burn the skin, stripping the outer, older layers in order to expose the younger layers. This makes the skin look more supple and fresh. The problem, however, is that lasers use light of certain wavelengths to produce the heat that's used during the treatment. For many people of color, skin color is so close to the color of their hair and blood vessels in terms of wavelength that the laser does not know which it is burning. If the skin absorbs too much heat, scarring can result. Dark skin is not the problem; it is our lack of technology at the present time. Research is being conducted on better light sources with wider wavelengths that can be pulsed to deliver a small amount of heat. In the future, such lasers may prove quite valuable for treating women of color.

-Part Two-

The Twenties

Most plastic surgery procedures address the concerns of aging. For that reason, I arranged this book in chronological order, starting with procedures that are viable in your twenties and working forward from there. Some of the common problems that aesthetic plastic surgery procedures address include the inability to lose unwanted pounds, protruding abdomen as a result of childbirth, drooping of the breasts due to gravity, jowling, furrowing of the brow, puffy eyes, and so on.

I personally believe that women shouldn't consider aesthetic procedures until they reach their twenties. Skeletal maturity has to be reached before surgery can be performed, unless there is some physical deformity that would affect psychological development. Also, without skeletal maturity, there is no way for the surgeon to predict results.

Nevertheless, with the pressures placed on women today, it is no wonder that many of you are considering procedures at younger and younger ages. From a psychological standpoint, it is legitimate that your concerns about your appearance be addressed.

7

Rhinoplasty (Nose Surgery)

I WANT TO SHARE with you the story of Natalie, a very wonderful little girl. She sent me a letter that read:

Hello Dr. Adams,

This letter really comes from the heart. I hope after reading it you can understand what I'm going through and be willing to help me out. The reason why I'm writing you is I need a really big favor. Well, I'll be fourteen soon, and next year I'm starting high school, which is one of the most important years of my life. I have very low self-esteem. I'm hoping that you can give me a nose job. Please, Dr. Adams, I know that's money and a big favor, but help me, please. I feel I can have a normal teenage life (by this surgery). I know I'm a minor but my mother is willing to sign a consent form or something, even though she doesn't agree with me in this surgery. I feel I should be fairly happy with my nose done, and what I'm feeling now is the worst. Dr. Adams, I really don't expect you to understand what I'm going through, but please be willing to help me out.

Always,
Natalie

P.S., I pray that you can call me back during your lunch break, home, etc., and explain to me the pros and cons of having this surgery and mainly say you're willing to help me out. Thanks for your time and patience.

Natalie's letter had a big impact on me. I felt numb. I knew we needed to sit across from each other and discuss this. I had to help her work through the pain she was obviously feeling. Puberty is unkind to all adolescents, but thinking of a nose job at fourteen seemed irrational to me. There were so many other more important things she could be focusing on at this time. How wrong I was. In today's world, that's exactly what teens think about. They think about looks, clothes, music, and the opposite sex. To be honest, I guess I did, too, when I was that age.

I called Natalie the following day. In my most professional doctor voice, I encouraged her to come in for a consultation. I asked that she bring her mother, but I also made it a point not to sound judgmental. As I entered the exam room, her mother smiled almost apologetically, but it was easy to see that she was relieved.

"Hello, Dr. Adams," they replied in unison.

I was direct. I turned to the mother and asked if she'd had an opportunity to read Natalie's letter.

"Yes," she said, nodding. "I had no idea that she was feeling like this, nor did I realize she felt so strongly." Natalie sat quietly, avoiding eye contact, but her manner was relaxed. She had carried these feelings around for so long that I guess it was a relief just to get them off her chest.

When I asked Natalie to tell me about her problem, tears began to well up in her eyes. "It's my nose," she said. "I hate it."

"What do you mean, you hate it?" I asked. "What do you hate about it?"

"I don't like it here." She pointed to her nostrils. "I just don't like it."

I explained to Natalie that she would have to be a little more specific if she wanted me to help. So far she'd told me nothing. I needed specifics. I have to be able to say, OK, this is what she's complaining about, and that represents an anatomic structure that I can change.

I paused to allow Natalie time to collect herself. Then I asked her to try to explain her problems with her nose again. This time I suggested that she pretend that her mother and I were not here. I wanted her to look in the handheld mirror, as if she were alone, and talk out loud about the kinds of things she felt were wrong with her nose.

"Well, for one, it's too wide," she began tentatively. "When I smile in pictures, it covers half my face." I nodded encouragingly. "And here," she continued, "The top is too flat. I don't like right here at the tip. It's like a ball. I just don't like any of it."

That was the kind of feedback I needed. I thanked her and then I explained how I, as a surgeon, looked at noses. I suggested that she keep looking in the handheld mirror so that she could see what I was talking about. I asked her to sit up tall.

"When I look at noses," I explained, "I start at the hairline. The distance from the hairline to the root of the nose, the nasion, should equal the length from the nasion to the base of the columella, the point in the center of the nose where the nose attaches to the lip; and that in turn should equal the distance from the columella to the chin. In a sense, the face should be divided into thirds, and each third should be pretty much the size of the nose.

"If you look at the side of the face in a profile and hold your head in what is called a Frankfurt horizontal, which is with a line drawn from the eyes to the ear parallel to the floor, then a line drawn straight down from where the columella meets the lips should hit the tip of the chin. If the chin is behind this line, it's too short. If it's in front of this line, it's too large. A lot of times people come in complaining that their nose is too big when it's really their chin that's too small.

"Now, the nose can also be divided into thirds. If you feel the top of the nose and start coming down toward the tip, you'll feel a ledge. This ledge is where the bones of the nose end. This is the upper third of the nose. The middle third of the nose is formed by the upper

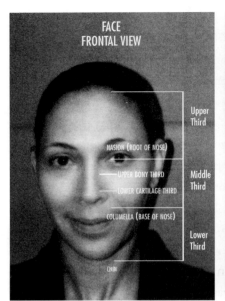
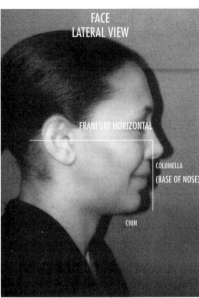

Figure 5: From an aesthetic and geometric standpoint, the face can be divided into thirds. In the frontal view, the diagram from the hairline to the root of the nose should equal the length of the nose, which in turn should equal the distance from the columella to the chin. In other words, the nose divides the face into thirds.

In the lateral view with the head held in the Frankfurt Horizontal, a perpendicular line dropped from the columella should connect to the chin. If the chin sits behind this line, it may not be the nose that is too large, but the chin that is too small. If the chin sits in front of this line, it may be that the nose isn't small, but that the chin is too big.

lateral cartilages, and the bottom third is formed by what's called the alar cartilages, which are the cartilages that form the rim of the nostrils. I mention these structures, Natalie, because it is these structures under the skin that determine, to a certain extent, how your nose looks. The skin is really just a cover that conforms to the shape of these bones and cartilages.

"You described three common complaints that people have about their noses, and each is easy enough from a surgical standpoint to address. For one, you feel that the top is too flat; this can be addressed by taking cartilage from inside the nose and placing it on top of the bones in the upper third of the nose. Of course, the cartilage is placed under the skin.

"Your description of the tip looking like a ball is also quite accurate. This is addressed by sculpting the top of the alar cartilages. The ala, including the outside rim of skin, will also have to be trimmed to narrow the nose so that when you smile it doesn't cover half your face."

Natalie nodded in agreement at the proposed changes, but I knew that there was another issue contributing to Natalie's problem that we needed to discuss. She said she "hated" her nose. We needed to explore why. So I asked Natalie how she would describe the perfect nose.

She paused, looking a bit blank, and then said, "I don't know. I just don't like this one. I don't like how big it is." Natalie couldn't— or wouldn't—answer my question.

In plastic surgery, we're always talking about aesthetics. The word *aesthetics* originally referred to people's ability to see things around them. Today it has come to mean beautiful or pleasing. But beauty is in the eye of the beholder.

"Let's face it," I told her. "You and I are black. When we look in magazines, we see mainly white faces. Our popular culture has told us that these people represent beauty. To be specific, though, our American notion of beauty has really been borrowed—or stolen— from the ancient Greeks. Our cultural ideal can be seen in the faces on statues such as the Apollo Belvedere or Venus de Milo."

Natalie nodded. "I've seen them in books," she said.

"Those faces have noses where the root is in the same plane as the forehead. A natural, uninterrupted curve extends from the eyebrows to the lateral aspects of the nose. The nose itself is long and narrow, with nostrils that are long and thin. The cheeks, even though they are high, are not too pronounced. They curve gently to define a hollow at the level of the mouth that is connected to a strong, well-defined, square chin. This is the face that you see on a lot of models."

The reason I was explaining this, I told Natalie, was that this facial ideal created a lot of problems and unhappiness for *white* Amer-
icans who didn't look like those statues. So I wanted her to imagine
how ridiculous it was for us to emulate it. I know a lot of plastic surgeons who have tried to put this nose and this chin on black faces. It
just doesn't fit. We have all seen performers with this nose. I'm not
going to mention names, but we all agree something just isn't quite
right.

I wanted Natalie to realize that yes, it was reasonable for her to
want to improve her appearance. It was also reasonable for her to want
some balance in her face. No feature, be it your nose, your lips, or
your chin, should overshadow any other feature of your face. But it
was not reasonable for her to want the Venus de Milo's nose. Natalie's
nose should fit in with the rest of her face.

But she also needed to think about the fact that her nose is not on
her face only to look good. It also has to allow her to breathe. When
we talk about changing the structure of the nose, we also have to
take into consideration how it functions. Making it too narrow can
make it difficult to breathe. The nose is really a pyramid and not just
simply a triangle. If I do something to one side, it affects the other
side. As a surgeon, I have to take into consideration that if you have a
large hump on your nose and I shave that down, the tip will come up.
If your tip is already tilted up and I shave down the dorsum, or top of
the nose, as the tip rotates up further, you'll practically be able to see
into your brain. The point is, if you do something in one area you
generally need to compensate in another. So there are a number of
things you have to consider when you start to talk about nose surgery.

Natalie seemed to get the message, so we went back to discussing
her nose and what could be done about it. For her, it was a good-
news-bad-news situation. The good news was that I agreed her nose
was a bit large for her face. It would be reasonable to elevate the tip
and better define it. It would also be reasonable to remove some of

the flaring of the nostrils. The dorsum could also come up, either by augmentation, which is onlaying bone or cartilage, or by breaking the bones and moving them in.

The bad news, though, was that Natalie wasn't physically ready for the surgery. At fourteen, she hadn't completely finished growing. I made it clear that she would be a good candidate for rhinoplasty, but that she shouldn't have the surgery yet. I wasn't putting her off; the timing of surgery is extremely important. Skeletal maturity is absolutely necessary in order to get a result that's predictable. I hoped Natalie would take my advice and drop the notion of surgery at this time, but I continued the consultation as if she wouldn't. I figured it was good for her to know exactly what she would experience when—and if—she had the procedure done.

Natalie was somewhat teary-eyed, but it was obvious that she was paying close attention. She seemed relieved to at least have her concerns addressed.

I told her that during a rhinoplasty, I use general anesthesia. I want surgery to be a pleasant and pain-free experience. With general anesthesia, you go to sleep with a problem and you wake up with it solved. Some people ask to use local anesthesia instead, and that's reasonable, even though I don't recommend it. I find that people have a better experience if they don't have to deal with the trauma of me working on their face while they're awake.

The operation itself takes about two hours. It depends on what needs to be done, and there are a number of things to consider. For example, a bump on your nose can be removed either by chipping off some of the bone using a chisel called an osteotome, or it can be removed by gentle sanding. The determining factor is really how much bone needs to be removed. The cartilage at the tip of the nose can be contoured to give a nice projection of the tip. Some irregularities of the nose can be smoothed by adding cartilage taken from the septum—the wall between the nasal cavities. If the nostrils are too wide, they can be narrowed by removing a small pie shape from the side crease. In some patients who have problems breathing, an adequate airway can be created either by straightening a deviated septum or reducing the size of the nasal turbinates. The nasal turbinates are folds of skin and bone inside the nose that function to humidify, moisturize, and warm the air we breathe.

First of all, I told Natalie and her mother, it's important to watch for signs of a respiratory infection or a cold in the days before surgery. If you get sick, call the office; we may have to reschedule your procedure until you're healthy. The night before and the morning of surgery, you'll need to wash your face, neck, and ears with an antibacterial soap. Shampoo your hair, but don't style it. Most important, don't put on makeup prior to coming to the surgery center. Wear comfortable, loose-fitting clothes and flat shoes that are easy to put on. If there are any medications that you take regularly, take those the morning of surgery with sips of water. But don't eat breakfast. Make sure you have somebody lined up to stay with you the night after the surgery.

The operation itself is pretty straightforward once we have a plan. You will arrive at the surgery center about an hour to an hour and a half before the procedure is to be done. At that time, you meet the anesthesiologist, whom you've certainly talked with the night before. He or she goes over your medical history and asks a lot of questions that you've probably already answered. Don't get annoyed. For my money, the most important issue in plastic surgery is safety. Your medical information is double-checked to make sure that everything is covered.

Then the anesthesiologist puts in your intravenous line. The intravenous line is there to give you fluids and medicines while you're asleep. Before we begin surgery, you will be given some antibiotics. Then we will take you into the operating room, where the procedure will occur. When we're finished with the surgery, you'll be brought back to the recovery room. You'll stay there for about two hours. During this time the anesthesia wears off and you'll become fully awake. There will be light packing in your nose. If we have moved the bones on the top or side of the dorsum of the nose, you will have a plaster or plastic splint on your nose for protection. The splint is just a cast to hold the bones in place while they heal.

Following surgery, there will be some oozing from your nose. This is normal and lasts for at least a day or two. A bandage called a sniffer will have been placed over the nostrils to catch this flow. Try not to swallow any blood, because it can cause nausea. Gently spit it out.

On the second and third day after surgery, gently clean your nostrils with peroxide. This helps remove crusted blood and keeps the incision lines clean. By day three after surgery, I'd like you to wash your nose with plain old soap and water two to three times a day. The best antibiotic we've come up with is still soap and water. Then put Bacitracin or Neosporin ointment on the incision line. Neosporin is an antibacterial ointment, but I don't use it for that purpose. What I want to do is keep any bleeding that occurs along the suture line moist so that it can easily be washed off. What we're trying to do is prevent any of that hard crusting. Remember when your grandmother said, Don't pick that scab? Well, she was 100 percent wrong. Crusting causes increased inflammation and therefore increased collagen deposition. This leads to more scarring. The cleaner you can keep that incision line, the better, regardless of how you do it. I prefer you to wash it. Some people like to pick it.

After surgery, I generally give patients an antibiotic to take orally for about five days and pain medicine to take for about three to five. Most people who have nose surgery tell me they don't really have pain. You may feel stuffy, as if you need to blow your nose. However, I ask that you *don't* blow your nose. Also, you may have to mouth-breathe for a short time due to nasal packing. Bear with this for a day or two, but more important, avoid activities that can lead to coughing or sneezing.

It takes about five to seven days to feel pretty much back to normal. This is the worst you'll go through, in my opinion. If you bend over, lift something heavy, or blow your nose, you increase the venous pressure, and this could lead to bleeding. For most people who have serious bleeding after nose surgery, the problem doesn't start until about a week after surgery, when they start to feel good. So this is the time when you must be more careful. I repeat: *Don't blow your nose.*

I'll see you two days after surgery to take out the packing. I'll see you again five to seven days postoperatively to remove the sutures, and again at about two weeks postop to remove the splints. After three weeks you'll be able to go back to your regular life. I ask that you slowly resume your normal activities.

I finished my explanation of rhinoplasty. Then I told Natalie and her mother that I generally end the consultation at this point. They needed time to absorb the all the information. If they had further questions later, or wanted to pursue the surgery, we could schedule a second consultation.

A second consultation is necessary only for patients who are ready to go through with their surgery. During this visit, I answer questions and go over everything you'll need to know before surgery. I obtain any laboratory work we'll need. And we'll schedule the exact surgery date. We need at least three weeks notice prior to surgery in order to secure operating room time and make certain that we have adequate staffing. Before making a surgery date, patients need to think about things like vacation time, having adequate help around the house, transportation to and from the surgery center, and transportation to postoperative visits.

You'll need to pay for your surgery at the second consultation. Now, plastic surgery is expensive, and rhinoplasties, along with facelifts, are the most expensive procedures. The anesthesia can cost anywhere from $700 to $1,000. The operating room fee is about $1,500, and the surgeon's fee can run anywhere from $5,000 to $10,000. Yet even at that, in my opinion, it's clearly a bargain. Think about it. We spend $20,000 to $50,000 on a car that we drive for four years. Rhinoplasty is an investment in yourself, and it will be with you for the rest of your life

I asked if they had anything else they wanted to discuss at this point. They didn't have any questions, so Natalie's mom thanked me and they left. I'm not sure the fourteen-year-old was completely happy with what had taken place, but I hoped I had put things in proper perspective for her. I hoped that I had helped her by being honest. At any rate, I did not hear back from them.

Allison's Nasal Obstruction

Allison was a very shy twenty-two-year-old black female who came to the office complaining of nasal obstruction, difficulty breathing, and nasal congestion. She was a very beautiful, dark-skinned, petite woman who was 5'2" tall and weighed 108 pounds. Her skin was flawless and her face was thin and sculpted. Her forehead was prominent and her thick, curly hair was pulled back. Her chin and jaw were also prominent, and the combination of these two effects served to make her nose and mid-face seem short and wide.

Allison had just graduated from college and was starting her career as a speech pathologist. She was accompanied by her mother, who was a gynecologic nurse. I enjoyed watching them interact because it was obvious that they loved each other. More than that, it was clear that they were friends who had a tremendous amount of respect for each other. On examination, I saw that Allison had extremely large nostrils for her size and the size of her nose. Looking inside, it was easy to see why she complained of difficulty breathing. Her septum, the midline cartilage, was bowed in a C-shape and partially occluded both nostrils. The turbinate structures inside the nose, which warm and hydrate the air we breathe, were massively enlarged, contributing to the obstruction of the airway.

Allison had been complaining of obstruction of her right nostril with a history of coldlike symptoms for about a year. She had been using over-the-counter medications and nasal sprays for about six months without any relief. Her past medical history didn't reveal any problems. She had no known allergies.

She did, however, have her mother there, and her mother felt that if her daughter was going to undergo surgery, she was going to come out with the perfect nose for her face, both functionally and cosmetically. To their credit, they were quite specific about the changes they wanted. Allison did the talking, which was also encouraging. All too often, people present for surgery because of other people's reasons. She wanted her nostrils smaller, her tip more defined, and the dorsum longer and more prominent. She simply felt that her nose was too wide for her face.

From a functional standpoint, I suggested that we straighten out the septum inside her nose and reduce the size of her turbinates to make the airway larger. Cosmetically, she needed augmentation of the dorsum of the nose, along with a tip rhinoplasty and excision of the ala to narrow the nose.

We scheduled Allison for nasal septal reconstruction, submucosal turbinectomy bilaterally, and dorsal graft augmentation of the nose with a tip rhinoplasty, to be performed under general anesthesia. The morning of the surgery I examined her again. Another look at her laboratory values, including her blood count and urinalysis, demonstrated that they were all within normal limits. She was then taken to the operating room, where the anesthesiologist inserted her intravenous line. She was given IV fluids and antibiotics and gently put to sleep.

I performed the nasal septal reconstruction first. Restoring her ability to breathe freely was most important, and I did this by removing a piece of the septal cartilage, which separates the nostrils inside the nose. This resulted in the creation of airways on both sides, which allowed for the free passage of air.

I saved this cartilage to use to help raise the bridge of the nose. The skin was raised off the long cartilaginous structure of the nose. With the alar cartilages exposed, the top half of the cartilage was excised to get rid of the bulbous tip, to make it more sculpted. These cartilages, along with the septal cartilage, were then placed on the bridge of the nose to give it more height.

Finally, I removed small pie-shaped wedges from the outside rim of the nose to make it more narrow. The nose was then bandaged with a splint on the outside and gauze packing inside to provide gentle pressure, to prevent any bleeding.

Allison's postoperative course was unremarkable. I called her at home that evening to find out how she was doing. Her mother answered the phone. She said Allison was sleeping and appeared to be doing well. I assured her that I expected Allison to recover nicely, and I reminded her about the postop appointment in two days.

When they showed up for the office visit, I noticed that Allison's bandage was meticulous. Her mother, the nurse, had been taking good care of her. Allison was in fine spirits and even ventured a smile. Her biggest complaint was the packing in her nose, which was uncomfortable. The packing helps prevent any accumulation of blood. But the packing also makes it difficult to breathe. Breathing through your mouth can certainly keep you alive, but it isn't pleasant. It causes a foul taste in one's mouth and a foul smell to one's breath. I removed the packing, and Allison felt better immediately. I warned her, however, that she would still have to be careful. There was still the possibility of bleeding. And the nose was still quite fragile. What I wanted her to do was to return home and take it easy.

When Allison returned four days later, she was quite talkative and feeling well. She had begun to get ready for her new job and was

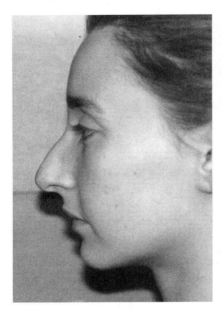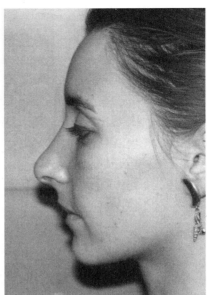

Figure 6: Rhinoplasty
Preop and postop photos of a 26-year-old female.

very optimistic. The splint on the dorsum of her nose had become loose because her postoperative swelling had gone down, so I removed it. I then gave Allison a mirror so she could examine her nose. I wanted her to see that the structure had been altered to make the changes that she felt were most important. I also took a nasal speculum and looked inside the nose to make sure that the incision lines were healing without problems. Everything looked fine.

I warned her that she was still in the danger period for bleeding. Her nose looked good and she wasn't in pain, but it was still possible to do damage. I asked that she not bend over and certainly not return to the gym for at least two more weeks. The body needs three weeks to recover before returning to such activities.

On her visit at three weeks postop, Allison was all smiles. She felt that the dorsum had been augmented to her satisfaction. She was concerned that her nostrils still looked a little large, but this would be resolved when the swelling went down. I emphasized that a pie-shaped area had been taken out of each nostril, and that even though they had been packed open, as the nose healed and the scars contracted, her nostrils would shrink.

It was good to see her smile, and I was happy that she was pleased with the results. I sat down to discuss with her the next two to three months. She was still feeling sort of tight and full in the nose area. I told her this was due to very minor swelling, which would go away over the next few months. We would take pictures at approximately three months postop, and compare them to the ones we took before surgery. Allison said she was extremely happy with the changes and felt that the surgery had been worth it. She gave me a hug.

8

Breast Augmentation

Chris: Desperately Seeking a C Cup

OFTEN WHEN I FIRST meet my patients, there is a bit of distance between us as they get a sense of who I am, while at the same time I'm
trying to find out exactly who they are. It's really all very normal, I
think, in terms of people's interpersonal reactions. It's natural to be
apprehensive about opening up with someone we really don't know.
In order to get patients where they are comfortable, I share up front
the things that I think are most important.

- · **Safety** is my first priority. Things should be planned well,
  the surgery should be flawless, and the patient should be
  back to his or her normal routine as quickly as possible.
- · **Surgery should be tailored to the individual.** Every
  operation should be designed specifically for the patient
  involved. In fact, I tell my patients that if a surgeon says
  this is *the* way I do it, run for the door. What determines
  how you do it is the patient's needs and desires, not the
  surgeon's lack of training and imagination.

Chris and I didn't need to go through the process of sizing each
other up. I had known her for six years. She had gone to school at
Wellesley College in Wellesley, Massachusetts, after having attended
prep school in New York. She was dating a close friend of mine, and
frankly, she knew more about me than I cared to admit.

Chris was a fair-skinned black woman with a lean, muscular body. At 5'10", she presented quite an imposing figure. She also was a slave to the gym, which balanced her propensity to party, and party she did. She was 127 pounds of almost pure muscle, which explained why she was flat-chested and otherwise fixated on her breasts. She talked constantly about having them augmented and now seemed ready to do it.

This is fairly common behavior. Many women go back and forth with friends and family about what they think is wrong with their appearance and what they would like done to improve it. When they finally decide to have the surgery, they want it done yesterday.

Chris wore a 34A bra and desperately wanted to be a C cup. I took the opportunity to explore her past medical and family history. During the physical exam, I estimated her breast volume to be approximately 150 cubic centimeters. This is done by comparing the breast volume present on the patient, to different sizes of implants. At twenty-six, Chris was exactly the right age to consider this operation. She had certainly reached skeletal maturity.

The Implant Controversy

Because I knew Chris, it was easy to discuss the breast implant controversy with blunt honesty. This is an issue that is impossible to ignore. I began by giving Chris my take on the things. First and foremost, I told her, understand that this whole thing has nothing to do with science. It's doctors versus lawyers, and, like 99 percent of the controversies in America, it's all about money.

I explained that the controversy got started when a reporter wrote an exposé about three women who argued that they developed autoimmune disease, a condition in which the body's defense system attacks itself, as a result of silicone breast implants. Never mind that two of the women had been diagnosed with autoimmune disease before they got their implants; that was merely a technicality that was omitted. Nevertheless, this reporter's haste was instrumental in persuading the wolves at the Lawyers Association of America to get involved. I know that every controversy requires at least two sides, and this issue was no different. Plastic surgeons have been implanting these devices for over thirty years, and yet no one had enough data to resolve the issue. I have to believe that this neglect was inspired by greed. Plastic surgeons were making $5,000 to $7,000 a procedure for placement of implants. It was money now, safety later, and worse yet, money now, information later. The conduct of the implant manufacturers was no better. Internal memos demonstrated that executives withheld information concerning the implants. This ranged from minor details like ignoring some of the problems women were having with them to covering up flaws in design.

However, there is no data whatsoever to support the conclusion that silicone gel breast implants cause autoimmune disease. Nevertheless, the end result was that saline implants would be used in the U.S. rather than silicone. It is important, however, to stress that when we refer to saline versus silicone implants, we are really talking about the material used to fill the implant. All implants are composed of a silicone shell. We recognize that silicone is relatively nonreactive in the body, and devices like catheters to infuse fluids and nutrients, penile prostheses, pacemakers, and knee and hip replacement parts are made of silicone.

The difference in the two really has to do with the feel of the implant under the skin. Silicone gel feels more like the body's subcutaneous tissue. Saline, or salt water, is heavier, more fluid, and gives the implant a harder feel.

I brought out an implant so that Chris could examine it as we discussed her surgery. This particular one was made by the McGann Company. There are other manufacturers, including a company called Mentor whose implants I also use occasionally. I asked Chris to

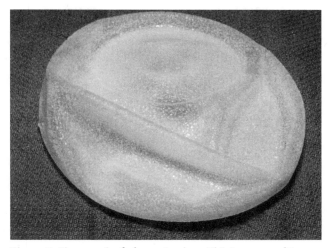

Figure 7: Photograph of a breast implant. This is a textured implant, which means its outer surface is rough to prevent capsular contracture.

feel the implant. She noted that the outside was rough and bumpy. I explained that this is a textured implant. Textured implants were designed to address one specific problem: capsular contracture.

Capsular Contracture

One of the known complications of implantation is capsular contracture, which is when hard scar tissue surrounds the implant once it's placed in the body. Any time you place a foreign object or implant in the body, the human body responds by forming a scar around it. In the case of implants, if the scar is thin and flimsy, it doesn't present a problem. However, if it's thick and hard, it does. With capsular contracture, you can see the implant as a round ball under the chest. It does not look or feel natural, like a breast. If the scar continues to contract and tighten around the implant, it can also result in pain. Unfortunately, there is no test to determine who will develop capsular contracture, and it is even more difficult to explain why some women get it on only one side when the surgery is done at the same time by the same surgeon. I personally feel that the formation of the capsule is related to things like bleeding, infection, bacterial contamination of the pocket, and also how the patient heals. Any one of these alone is able to cause the problem.

Capsular contracture led to the development of the textured implant. The scar, or capsule, causes problems when it is organized and regular. The fibers of the scar created by smooth implants were regularly aligned. As they contracted, they were able to squeeze down on the implant as a unit. The textured implant, with its rough outer shell, doesn't allow the scar fibers to align themselves regularly. They pull in different directions and negate each other. This reduces the likelihood of a hard, firm capsular contraction.

Above or Below the Muscle

The textured implant controversy also indirectly resolved another problem. A great deal of discussion goes into whether an implant should be placed above or below the muscle. Early studies demonstrated that when smooth implants were placed below the muscle, there was a lesser incidence of capsular contracture. So immediately we all began using submuscular placement. The rationale was that the tissue responsible for the formation of the thick scar was in the superficial fatty layer above the muscle. By placing the implant under the muscle, you avoided this interaction.

The problem, however, is that the normal breast sits on top of the muscle. There is no doubt that the best-looking augmented breast is one in which the implant sits on top of the muscle in its anatomic position. A problem, however, can exist in very thin women whose skin envelope cover does not allow for hiding the implant. In such cases, the imprint can be seen through the skin. The textured implant, with its irregularly arranged surface, also allows for the option of placing the implant in the space above the muscle.

I take another approach. What determines whether I place the implant above or below the muscle is the amount of soft tissue overlying it. I want the breast shape to be natural and the outline of the implant to be hidden. This depends in part on how much breast and subcutaneous tissue the patient has. Again, if the patient is thin, I put it below the muscle. If she has ample breast tissue or subcutaneous fat, I place the implant on top of the muscle.

Another technique I use is to split the pectoralis muscle, which is the large chest muscle. Thin women who have some ptosis, or drooping of the breast, from having had children previously get an excellent result with this technique. By splitting the muscle below the level of the nipple, the implant can be placed above the muscle in the lower quadrants, which gives the breasts a natural hang and a natural contour. The top half of the muscle is used to cover the top half of the implant, and this hides the implant and gives the breasts a natural conical shape.

It should be noted that placing the implant either below the muscle or above the muscle or splitting the muscle does not in any way affect one's ability to exercise or move the upper extremity. All three, however, require that you take it easy for approximately three weeks after surgery.

Incisions

Breast augmentation surgery normally takes about two hours. There are three different types of incisions that are used for placing the implants. The incision used is determined by the patient's need, preference, and body type, along with the surgeon's preference. The incision under the arm, though requested quite often, really works best for patients that have a very flat breast mound with minimal tissue. The attachment of the pectoralis muscle to the arm is used as a guide for placement, since the dissection is done very deep in this muscle without using direct vision.

The most common type of incision made is the inframammary incision, underneath the breast. It allows for dissection of an ample pocket and control of bleeding. However, the skin here is thick, and the tension on the incision from the weight of the implant can leave a most unfavorable scar.

Oddly enough, the best incision, and the one that took me the longest time to appreciate, is the circumareolar incision, around the nipple areolar complex. Intuitively, you'd think that an incision placed here would be easy to see because it's right up front at the most prominent part of the breast. That certainly was my belief. The problem with that logic, however, is that it does not take into consideration how we see. We see in borders and edges. We see as a result of contrast. By placing the incision just outside the areola, we can use the contrast between the areolar skin and the skin of the surrounding breast to hide the incision line.

I placed my hand in front of Chris with the dorsum, or back, facing outward on my left hand and my palm facing outward on the right. What I was attempting to show her was that we really see the borders of the dark side of the hand against the light side of the palm. The color change from the darker areola to the lighter surrounding skin allows for the incision line to be hidden or camouflaged. The incision is placed just outside the nipple areolar complex at the junction of the darker areola skin with the skin of the breast. This incision also allows for better access to the surgical field. An adequate pocket can be formed. It also allows for better control of bleeding, which helps prevent the formation of thick, hard scar tissue. Chris opted for the circumareolar incision. She had seen a number of girlfriends who had had augmentations and felt that would be the best scar for her. I agreed.

Once we decided on the placement of the incision, the next decision was the size of the implant. Most of the time, patients have a hard time saying what they would like their breasts to look like. Certainly, no one wants to appear as if they're trying to be so large that they become a cartoon character. An interesting study was done a few years back. Someone asked a hundred women to choose the ideal breasts out of a set of photographs. What was interesting was that the majority of them agreed on the same size. Regardless of whether a woman is 5 feet tall or 6 feet tall, the majority of women believe that a large C cup, conical in shape, is the ideal breast. This translates into a breast volume of between 400 and 450 ccs. So what I try to do is get you to that volume during breast augmentation. If I estimate that your breast volume is 100 ccs, then I place an implant from 330 to 360 ccs. Other considerations in determining the ideal size are the patient's hip size, the size and shape of the torso, and the amount of skin available to accommodate the implant.

The procedure begins as all operations in plastic surgery begin, with the preoperative preparation. For patients less than forty years of age, I only require a blood count and urinalysis. Older individuals require additional tests like a chest X ray and an EKG. You will certainly have talked to the anesthesiologist the night before, and on the morning of surgery, you two will meet. You will go over your medical history. Then the anesthesiologist prepares you for surgery by placing an intravenous line and giving you antibiotics and fluid intravenously. The preoperative markings, showing where I'll make the incisions, will be completed prior to taking you to the operating room.

Once in the operating room, you will be placed on your back on the operating room table with your arms out at about 90 degrees. The anesthesiologist will put you gently to sleep. The nursing staff will then wash your neck, chest, upper arms, and abdomen with a Betadine soap solution and then paint them with a Betadine paint solution that is an antibacterial agent. Sterile drapes will then be applied to the operative field. Because the implants are a foreign body, sterility is of the utmost importance.

The Operation

I use a small scalpel blade to make an incision around the nipple that cuts down through the skin to the level of the subcutaneous fat. A flap of skin is then raised to the level of the nipple. The incision is then taken straight down to the chest wall, dissecting through the subcutaneous tissue and breast tissue, using electrocautery. Electrocautery is a device much like a scalpel that uses electric current to dissect and cut tissue. The advantage of using electrocautery is that it also helps to minimize bleeding. Once the dissection has been carried down to the chest wall, a pocket is made for the implant on top of the muscle in the lower half of the breast. I often suggest that people think of a cross being drawn on the breast with its center at the nipple. The upper quadrants lie above the nipple, while the lower quadrants lie below. The pocket is extended to approximately 1 cm below the inframammary line so that the implants will sit properly. At the level of the nipple, I once again use electrocautery to transect the pectoralis major muscle. Using my hand, I form a pocket behind the muscle and on top of the rib cage. The pocket is then irrigated with normal saline to remove any loose tissue or fat. Again, we use electrocautery to stop any bleeding. Lap sponges, which are cloth gauze pads used to soak up excess blood and fluid, are then used to pack inside the pocket and to cover the wound. I do this to guarantee that all bleeding in the pocket is controlled before implant placement.

I then turn my attention to the other breast and repeat the process. The instruments are cleaned or changed, and the surgeon's gloves are changed to protect against contaminating the implants with bacteria. The implants are then opened and immediately placed in their pockets, care being taken to touch them as little as possible. The implants are inflated using normal saline, and the wounds are closed in three layers. The deep tissues are closed using Vicryl sutures, which dissolve, and the skin is closed using interrupted nylon sutures. However, many times what I try to do is close the wound without any sutures on the skin so that there is no chance of suture marks at a later time, after the wound has healed. This is done by placing dissolvable sutures just below the skin and using Steri-strips, or tape, to hold the wound edges together for five to seven days.

The final dressing consists of either Neosporin or Bacitracin ointment and a Xeroform gauze applied to prevent the dressing from sticking to the wound. This is all covered with gauze fluff and a thick, absorbent pad. Finally, the chest is wrapped with a couple of six-inch Ace bandages for comfort. You are then taken to the recovery room. Here I prescribe another dose of antibiotics, and you are kept in bed until you are fully awake and able to ambulate. You'll be given five days of antibiotics to take orally and from five to seven days' worth of pain medication. At that time, you can be taken home by whoever has accompanied you to the surgery center.

Postoperatively, Chris was seen two days after the surgery to make sure everything was okay. I generally wait two days because by that time the anesthesia has worn off, any nausea associated with anesthesia is over, and, frankly, patients complain less. At five to seven days postop, you will be brought back, and I remove any sutures that need to be taken out. I ask that you don't lift anything heavier than the telephone for the first three weeks. The only thing that can really go wrong at this time is infection, and by minimizing activity, we can minimize this complication. At three weeks, you can start back gradually to your regular activities.

People often ask about taking showers. Two days postoperatively, you can shower normally. You can also wear an athletic bra for the three weeks of healing time. I find that the initial bandage works well for the first forty-eight hours, and then afterward wearing an athletic bra both provides comfort and allows for easy removal when taking a shower or washing the incision lines.

Chris's postoperative course was uneventful. She was, however, quite dramatic and complained constantly of pain. By contrast, most people say their pain is not all that bad. However, by about the fifth to seventh day postoperative, she was happy and moving around comfortably, and getting back to her old self.

Chris, as with every patient, was also concerned about the longevity of her implants. My feeling is that they should last a lifetime with no particular hitch. The presence of an implant does not stop the aging process. And so, just like women who don't have them, with time, the breasts will begin to sag or droop. When this drooping becomes an issue, one may require a second procedure, the breast lift.

Complications

- **Bleeding:** Avoidance of this complication requires meticulous hemostasis (stopping bleeding) on the part of the surgeon and avoidance of aspirin-containing products on the part of the patient. Any medical illnesses (i.e., high blood pressure) should also be addressed.
- **Infection:** Can happen in 2 to 3 percent of cases. Avoidance requires strict adherence to surgical technique.
- **Capsular contracture:** Can result as a consequence of bleeding, infection, or the way the patient heals. Should

it occur, therapy may require re-operation to remove the thick scar.

· **Asymmetry:** A technical problem that should be addressed by the surgeon. May result from malposition or subsequent movement of an implant.

Cost

The final issue, which is certainly an important one, is price. The cost of anesthesia for the procedure is approximately $800. The implants themselves run around $1,200. The operating room fee is from $1,200 to $1,500, so even before we pay the surgeon, we're al-

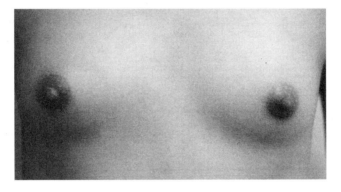

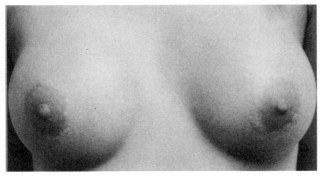

Figure 8: Pre- and postoperative augmentation mammoplasty in a 26-year-old female.

ready talking about $3,000. The surgeon's fee is approximately $4,000, making the surgery somewhere around $7,000. Nevertheless, in today's world, with competition running so high, you can probably get it done for less. But $7,000 is a realistic price.

When choosing a surgeon, don't go by price alone. Here are the kinds of things you should discuss with any doctor you are considering for your surgery:

1. How many of these procedures has your doctor done before?
2. Has your doctor had any complications, and if so, what was done about them?
3. Ask to see examples of your doctor's work. Look at photographs of the procedure done on other patients.
4. Ask to talk with other patients about their experience with this doctor.
5. Know how large you would like your breasts to be. Again, a very good rule of thumb is to aim for a large C cup (volume of approximately 450 ccs). This should include both the volume that you have plus the volume of the implant.

9

Reduction Mammoplasty

Melinda's Pain in the Neck

MELINDA CAME INTO THE office complaining of back and shoulder pain. I had treated her once before when she was a child for a small laceration that she had sustained while playing ball. Now she was twenty years old. Her current problem began at puberty, when her breasts developed to a size 34DD. Since she was 5'8" and 135 pounds, they were simply too large for her to tolerate. In the beginning they were merely a nuisance, interfering occasionally with her ability to perform in sports. Now the problem had progressed to the point where she was in constant pain. She'd had enough and was ready to do something about it.

When I entered the room, I told Melinda that she had certainly grown up.

"It was bound to happen," she snapped back.

"Smart, aren't we?" I said. Then I asked her to tell me what was going on. While she talked, I sat and admired this beautiful young woman whom I hadn't seen in quite a while. She was an elegant, bronze-colored black woman who demonstrated a presence that was clearly beyond her years. She was confident.

"Well, you see, Dr. Adams," she began, "I'm twenty years old now and in college. I go to Clark in Atlanta. I'm doing pretty well. I came in today to talk to you about my breasts. I'm interested in a reduction."

I nodded and explained that before we got started, I needed to catch up on her medical history since I'd last seen her.

Safety is the key to plastic surgery. Regardless of whether the surgeon has seen the patient before or not, a current, detailed medical history is of the utmost importance. Here are some of the questions I had for Melinda. You should know the answers to these questions before you go to your plastic surgery consultation.

- Do you have any medical illnesses that you need to see the doctor for? For example, things like asthma, heart disease, cancer, or diabetes.
- Does anyone in your family have any of the above medical problems?
- Does anyone in your family have breast cancer? Your mother, grandmother, or your sisters?
- Are you allergic to any medications?
- Do you have a history of bleeding or clotting problems? Do you bump yourself and bruise easily?
- Are you currently taking any aspirin or medications containing aspirin?
- Do you do breast self-exams? Do you ever feel lumps when you're doing the exam?
- Have you ever been pregnant?

Melinda looked at me indignantly before answering "no" to the last question. Otherwise she seemed confident as she searched the data banks of her brain for answers. Her medical history was normal.

We talked a bit more about the importance of breast self-exams and I applauded her for doing them every month. Breast disease, in particular breast cancer, is something that women ought to pay more attention to. Diseases like AIDS and Alzheimer's certainly attract more attention, but breast cancer affects more women on a personal level. *Everyone should learn to do breast self-exams. This can go far toward early detection, and early detection is the key to surviving breast cancer.* We really haven't improved on the survival rates for breast cancer in the past fifty years. Since the 1930s the average survival rate has remained at five years. A breast reduction is the ultimate breast biopsy, at least in terms of obtaining tissue for pathologic evaluation. If there is a tumor there, the reduction will surely get it out.

I asked Melinda what had made her decide to do something about her breasts now.

"I've been thinking about it for a while, Dr. Adams. I'm playing basketball and softball at school. At first when my breasts started getting large, it was just a nuisance. They were in the way when I tried to shoot baskets—just in the way all the time. I couldn't really do anything. Now I'm having pain in my back and shoulders and my breasts are so big that my bra straps dig into my shoulders."

All right, I told her. The next step was to get her in a gown and see what we could do to solve this problem. As we entered the exam room, I was struck by the fact that Melinda made me feel almost nostalgic. This time I was seeing her in my own office. I noticed that this exam room seemed different, much different, from the rooms that I had used in other surgeon's offices when I was just starting out.

This exam room is *me*. The emphasis is on warmth and comfort rather than the slick and the commercial. It is bright and inviting. In the center sits a 1938 Ritter Motor dental chair. It's gray with silver chrome, black armrests, and a footstool covered in black rubber. The hydraulics are in the front and raise the seat of the chair with a smooth, easy glide. The backrest requires manual elevation, but this makes for a more intimate relationship with the patient. I love that chair. Surrounding it are an antique reflecting light, a tin garbage can, and a classic Mayo stand, which is a metal table on wheels. A large floor-to-ceiling mirror is on the wall to the right of the chair. The other walls are covered with posters from early movies, including

Call It Murder with Humphrey Bogart. There is a round wooden table with two matching chairs in the corner in front of the examination chair. Behind the chair are cabinets that contain my supplies.

I allowed Melinda to change in the room alone, and I knocked before reentering to conduct my examination.

"Come in," I heard from behind the door. For the first time in a long time, I felt uneasy alone with a patient. The realization that this kid had grown up was sobering, and I wanted to afford her every courtesy due a grown woman.

The first thing I asked her to do was to stand up straight in front of the mirror. Her breasts were large and pendulous. The bulk of tissue extended down below the mammary folds. The nipples were large and extended below this reference line also. Indeed, her breasts had begun to infringe upon her waistline, making her abdomen look prominent when in fact it wasn't. I measured the suprasternal notch to nipple distance for each breast. This was an indication of just how much drooping, or ptosis, she had. It was 27 cm on the right and 25.5 cm on the left. I jotted this down in her chart.

I proceeded methodically with my exam. When I finished, I asked if she had any questions for me.

"Yeah, a few," she offered.

I told her I'd be happy to answer them. But first, she could get dressed and meet me in my office. We would go over everything there.

After a few minutes, there was a knock at my door and I called for Melinda to come in and take a seat. To start with, I told her she was a perfect candidate for a reduction. As I noted in the exam, her suprasternal notch to nipple distance was 27 cm on the right and 25.5 cm on the left. Normal for someone her age who hasn't had any children is somewhere between 18 and 21 cms.

I explained that it's of little consequence that the nipples are different distances on each side. They are in everybody. We're two-sided animals, and no one's sides match. I wanted her to notice this now, preoperatively. During the procedure I would make Melinda's breasts equal, but I wanted her to understand that they weren't equal from the start. Postoperatively, people stare at themselves and get a little crazy about perfection. Nobody is perfect, but I do my best to get my patients as close to perfection as possible.

There are a number of procedures that can be used to reduce the size of breasts:

- *Amputation.* The earliest procedures involved simple amputation of the breasts. The breast is cut off at the appropriate level and the nipple is transposed, or moved, as a free graft, much like a skin graft.
- *Standard Wise pattern reduction.* In this procedure, the nipple is raised, supported by a bridge of skin and subcutaneous tissue called a pedicle. The tissue on either side of this bridge is excised, sort of like cutting a pie. The nipple is moved or transposed based on an inferiorly anchored pedicle consisting of breast tissue and skin, which allows for the formation of a normal conical shape of the breast. This also preserves nipple sensation.
- *Minimal scar techniques.* These procedures use some variation of the Wise pattern and generally attempt to omit the horizontal limb of the scar.
- *Bennelli technique.* Used most often in those women requiring only a minimal lift. The final scar is an incision around the areola and in selected patients gives an excellent result.

For Melinda, the standard inferior pedicle procedure was the best solution. It gives an excellent result, with a good shape to the breast. The downside is the resultant scar. You end up with a scar that's an inverted T, with a circular scar around the nipple areolar complex.

The scar around the nipple areolar complex is hidden fairly well because of the color differences between the areola and the surrounding skin. The lower limb, or the horizontal limb, of the T is hidden by the breast itself. It lies in the inframammary fold out of view. The only part of the scar that is visible is the vertical limb. It is in clear view and can be widened due to the weight of the breasts and the subsequent tension on the incision line.

Most women, however, gladly opt for the scars rather than the pain and humiliation of excessively large breasts. In fact, of all the surgeries we perform as plastic surgeons, breast reduction patients seem to be the happiest postoperatively. A few scars are much better than carrying around all that weight. It's certainly better to have scars that are hidden than to have people constantly staring at your breasts because they are so large, or even worse, to have constant shoulder and back pain.

Preoperative Planning

I told Melinda that the most important element for ensuring a good outcome to her surgery was the preoperative planning. Markings for surgery are done in the preoperative holding area prior to surgery, and in many respects this *is* the surgery. Once the markings are done, the surgery really involves connecting the dots.

You and I decide exactly how much breast tissue to take out and where to place the nipple. We begin by marking the midline of the chest. Then from the suprasternal notch, I design an equilateral triangle with the sides about 20 to 21 cm long. The apex of the triangle is the suprasternal notch, and the nipples form the corners of the triangle. Sometimes I give you stickers to help you determine at what level you want the nipple placed. After this is done, I draw the incisions. The pattern I use is called a Wise pattern, and Wise is one of the surgeons who helped develop the technique. The interesting

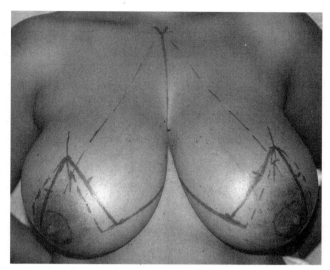

Figure 9: Wise pattern, preoperative markings for reduction mammoplasty in a 28-year-old female.

thing is, what he did was essentially flatten out a bra to help define where the incisions should go to reshape the breast as a cone. After the markings are complete, we're ready to go to the operating room.

I asked Melinda if she wanted to ask questions at this point.

"Not yet," she said. "Let me just hear the rest. I'm sure I'll have some questions later."

I continued my explanation of the procedure. "When we move into the operating room," I told her, "you're placed on your back on the operating room table. Then they paint your chest with a Betadine paint solution. When it dries, it's an effective antibacterial agent. That's how iodine works in killing bacteria. Then we drape you with sterile drapes to wall off the operative field. Draping is really just covering the body areas not involved in the surgery. First, I de-epitheliaize the skin pedicle. De-epitheliazation means cutting off the top layer of skin. The pedicle, if you remember, is the area that will hold the nipple. I'll leave the bottom layer of skin intact to give good blood supply to the nipple. I make the base of the pedicle about

10 cm wide. I also measure the nipple areolar complex and, if it's required, reduce it to make the areola approximately 38 mm in diameter. These numbers will have been figured out preoperatively and are based on what is considered standard for most breasts. After this is complete, pie sections of the breast tissue are removed to fashion the breasts as a cone. Flaps, which are layers of skin and fat, will then be dissected, with their thickness about $\frac{1}{4}$ to $\frac{1}{2}$ inch. The flaps are draped around this pedicle to form the conical breast. Just before we close the incisions, I'll put in a drain. A drain is a tube that's used to allow for the removal of fluid from the wound cavity. After a few days, I'll take this drain out. The rest of the procedure is just closing the wound and sewing the incisions.

"I'll see you a day or two after the operation. You'll have a bulky bandage on, so there's really nothing to see. What I'm checking is the amount of drainage from the wound. If there's quite a bit, then the drains will stay."

"How much is quite a bit?" Melinda interrupted.

I told her that 30 cc or so in eight hours would be considered "quite a bit." If it's much less than that, then we can take out the drains. This is just a check to make sure that things are going according to plan and to address any postoperative questions you might have. I'll see you five days later to take out sutures, and finally at about three weeks after the operation to get you started back to your regular activities. After that, we'll see each other at three months and then at six months, when we'll take "after" photos to compare with your "before" shots.

In Melinda's case, I would probably take off anywhere from 700 to 800 cc of tissue from each breast. To call it a breast reduction, a minimum of 500 cc needs to be removed. Anything less is considered a mastopexy, or breast lift, not a reduction. The distinction is important because in cases where less than 500 cc of tissue are removed from each breast, insurance companies have opted not to pay for the procedure, calling it cosmetic rather than reconstructive. Clearly, this wouldn't be a problem for Melinda.

Complications

It's always hard to talk about complications, but it's important to cover what could go wrong during surgery. My biggest worry is that this discussion unnecessarily scares people. It opens doors that probably don't need to be opened, but patients should know both the benefits and the risks of a procedure. Here are some of the possible complications of breast reduction surgery:

- *Devascularization of the nipple.* This is the most disastrous thing that can happen, at least in my mind, Devascularization is a loss of blood flow to the nipple. This leads to color changes in the areola or loss of the nipple itself.
- *Malpositioning of the nipple.* Malposition is when the nipple is placed too high, or not along the nipple mammary line. This is a major problem. Once tissue has been cut out, you can't put it back. The solution is adequate planning to make sure that this doesn't happen.
- *Inappropriate skin resection.* Either too much or too little skin is taken out. This makes the breasts look boxy or square.
- *Asymmetry.* Asymmetry refers to unevenness of size between the two breasts, or a discrepancy in their position on the chest wall. This is a technical error on the part of the surgeon and can be avoided by adequate planning.
- *Skin necrosis, fat necrosis.* This is a loss of tissue in the area where the horizontal and vertical limbs of the T incision come together. These are manifestations of inadequate blood flow.

In addition to these complications, there are other possible problems that aren't specific to breast reduction surgery. They include infection, bleeding, and hypertrophic scarring. Hypertrophic scarring refers to the thick, red, raised scars associated with dark skin. Hypertrophic scars are not keloids and can be corrected, but they are something to watch out for.

Melinda was looking far away, deep in thought. Her eyes blinked as she processed this information. I felt comfortable that she had retained the things I said, but I wanted to be sure. Finally, she spoke up. "I guess you've answered all my questions for the moment. I'm sure I'll think of plenty of others once I walk out the door."

I said that before she left, we should talk about cost, even though her insurance would probably cover at least part of it.

Cost of Breast Reduction Surgery

Breast reduction surgery is a long operation and can take anywhere from three to four hours. The fee for using the operating room for three and a half hours is around $1,800. The anesthesia fee is from $700 to $1,000, which makes the total $2,500 to $2,800 right off the bat. A reduction mammoplasty itself can run anywhere from $6,00 to $8,500 for the surgeon's fee. So you're looking at around $10,000 for this operation.

"Wow," Melinda said. "That is a lot of surgery."

I smiled. I added that there is also a lot of follow-up involved in this procedure. Patients have a lot of incisions and a lot of questions. Both mind and body require significant postoperative care. There will be dressing changes, drain removal, and general encouragement, because psychologically, reduction mammoplasty is a lot to deal with. I promised her I'd earn every penny of the fee.

Melinda underwent a reduction mammoplasty approximately one month later. Postoperatively there was some loss of tissue where the

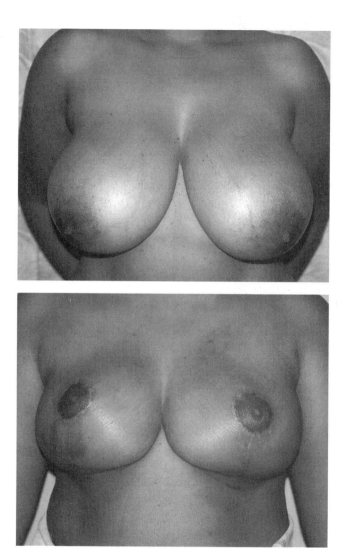

Figure 10: Pre- and postoperative photos of a reduction mammoplasty in a 26-year-old female.

horizontal and vertical limbs of the T-incision come together in the
inframammary fold. This was allowed to heal on its own, the only
therapy required being to wash the incision line twice a day with
soap and water, apply Neosporin ointment, and cover the wound
with a gauze sponge.

The horizontal, inframammary line incision was also thick and hypertrophic. I treated this with Kenalog to reduce the scarring. There was considerable improvement, but I personally continue to hate the scars in this procedure.

Melinda, however, was ecstatic. She no longer had bra straps digging into her shoulders, or the associated back and shoulder pain. She went back to college that fall a very happy woman.

-Part Three-

The Thirties

The thirties are a very interesting age for most women. Often they have settled into careers, childbearing has ended, and their focus is turning back to themselves. This is the time of life, however, when women begin to notice a few unflattering changes in their appearance. One problem is that childbearing has taken its toll. Another issue is that those fatty deposits that used to be a cinch to get rid of no longer respond to dieting or exercise. These are the years when many women start to consider rejuvenative plastic surgery to help them recapture their youthful figures. This section will focus on liposuction, mastopexy (breast lifts), and abdominoplasty (tummy tucks).

10

Suction-Assisted Lipectomy

Donna's New Contours

ONE DAY A LOVELY and charming woman named Donna showed up at my office. Her mannerisms were relaxed, but her speech suggested a sense of urgency. This is often the case when women in her age group—the mid-thirties—come in for rejuvenative surgery. In a sense, doctors get a view of people that is a photograph, a picture in time. It's hard to tell what was going on just before or just after that picture. All you see is the patient's state of mind at the moment they choose to come in for a consultation. I suspect that most patients agonize over the decision of whether to have a procedure long before they share their beliefs with someone else. By the time I see them, the decision has pretty much been made and they're ready to go. They don't really need convincing; they're just trying to get things scheduled before they change their mind. The purpose now is to become comfortable with the surgeon—that's it.

I could tell that there was a lot going on inside Donna. She was a woman in the midst of redefining her life. She was full of energy. She'd married early, had two children, gotten divorced, and then decided to continue her education. When I met her she was thirty-four years old and in the last year of law school. She looked somewhat mature, but her skin was flawless. She glowed. She was also planning to remarry in six months and she wanted to look as good as possible, not only in her dress but also on her honeymoon.

Donna began our consultation by insisting: "Dr. Adams, you've *got* to give me liposuction."

At first I was surprised, because she was quite thin. In fact, she was 5'9" and weighed only 140 pounds. But Donna had a problem that is common with women seeking liposuction—she had considerable saddlebagging of her lateral thighs. You could see it through her pants, and it was even more visible when she was in a dress. She was a great candidate for liposuction because her problem was an isolated pocket of fat in a woman who was otherwise thin. In her situation, the result would be absolutely fantastic and quite dramatic.

I asked her why she wanted liposuction at this point in her life.

"I've thought about it for a while," she said. "Up until I really started studying hard for the bar, I was working out a lot, but I have these areas I just can't get rid of. My trainer thinks I'm crazy. He says I should just lose weight to address the problem. I really want to know what you think. I really don't want to be any thinner. I've been considering getting my eyes done, too, but that can wait."

I agreed that getting her eyes done could wait. I was concerned that she was thinking about having surgery in the middle of studying for the bar exam. I asked her if it would be better to consider surgery after the exam was over. There will be a recovery period, I reminded her. It may only be three to six weeks, but that could be time well spent studying.

She nodded. "Yeah, I do, I need that time. But I've been studying a lot and I needed a rest. I thought I'd come over and get some information. You know, get started in terms of understanding what I need to do to get all this done before my wedding in six months. I certainly don't want to wait until the last minute. Besides, it's a good break from studying just to come in and talk."

I laughed. "Good for whom?" I wanted to know.

"Good for both of us, Dr. Adams. I get the scoop from you, and at the same time, you get to help me. I really want to ask you about this new ultrasound liposuction. You do that, don't you? It sounds kind of neat."

"Neat," I repeated.

"Yeah, neat, like a good idea. I mean, I don't know. You know better than me, so tell me about it."

I paused for a few seconds to collect my thoughts.

First, I told Donna, let's begin on the same page. Everyone who comes in has a different level of understanding of what liposuction really is. They've read some magazine or talked with a friend who's had it done, and they have a preconceived notion of what liposuction is all about. Regardless of what they have heard, though, I try to start at the beginning.

There are three things that make liposuction possible:

- **Fat cells.** Up until puberty (generally fourteen to sixteen in females and sixteen to eighteen in males), the body stores fat by increasing the number of fat cells. After puberty, the body stores fat by increasing the size of the fat cells that already exist. In other words, there is hyperplasia, or an increase in number, before puberty and hypertrophy, or the cells getting larger, after puberty.

- **Where fat is stored.** The body has a predilection for storing fat in certain locations. Men generally store fat in their abdomen and flanks—that spare tire look—while women tend to store fat in the lower abdomen and lateral thighs, the saddlebag deformity.

- **How fat is stored.** There is a tendency to store fat wherever we store it first and lose it there last. This stored fat persists regardless of diet or exercise. In some people, this area is the abdomen, while in others it's in their lateral thighs or hips.

Donna interrupted. "I can certainly attest to that," she said as she pinched her thighs.

I smiled. "Exactly," I said. "So when you put all those facts together, liposuction makes sense."

Liposuction Question Number One

Then, before she had a chance to ask, I answered the most commonly asked question in plastic surgery: *If I get liposuction, will the fat come back?* The real answer is yes and no, but mainly no, and I don't say that to be evasive. It's just that you have to consider a number of variables before you can say no unequivocally. If you believe the argument that after puberty the body does not increase the number of fat cells but only their size, then it's fair to say that the cells removed by liposuction are gone and they're never coming back. Now, I said *if* you believe that, because there are some researchers who don't. There was one study done on women that indicated that an increase in the number of fat cells as well as in their size occurs with weight gain. Other investigators argue that the hormones of pregnancy stimulate fat cells to divide. So it seems that during pregnancy, at least, women may be producing new fat cells. The jury is still out, so the issue is not completely resolved. One thing is certain: Whether there is an increase in the number of fat cells with weight gain or not, the primary deformity does not come back. You may gain weight or increase the amount of fat in your body, but the areas that have been suctioned do not get as large as they would have if liposuction had not taken place. In other words, the storage area for fat is smaller. Some people interpret this to mean that fat is just stored in a different area. I don't think that's true. Fat is a metabolic storage tissue that's stored throughout the body. Certainly it is stored in some areas more than others, but I think from a metabolic standpoint that we must consider the whole of stored fat as systemic, or throughout the body.

It's important to remember that *liposuction is a body contour procedure, not a weight loss procedure.* Liposuction removes strips of fat from the subcutaneous tissue, creating a series of tunnels in the subcutaneous fat. The areas where fat has been removed collapse upon themselves, resulting in the contour changes that, ideally, both the doctor and the patient were trying to achieve.

Liposuction itself is an easy procedure to do. That's why so many different types of doctors try to do it. But it's not an easy procedure to do *well.* Here's the best way I can explain liposuction: Imagine that a sponge is sitting on the kitchen sink. The sponge material represents the subcutaneous fat. What liposuction does is put the holes in the sponge. Now, when a sponge dries, it gets thinner as the holes collapse on each other. That's exactly analogous to wound healing. As your body heals, the areas where suctioning was done collapse on the spaces made by removal of the fat. This is what allows the surgeon to contour the body. By removing isolated areas of fat and paying attention to detail, the surgeon can smooth out the bulges caused by excess deposits of fat. What makes it difficult to do well is that it ultimately comes down to using a round tube to make a flat surface. This requires meticulous work and a lot of patience, and most people don't have that.

I paused to see if Donna had understood everything. She had.

"OK, then," I said. "Now I'll answer your first question. Ultrasonic liposuction is an attempt to take advantage of the fact that sound waves can liquefy fat, making it easier to remove the fat with suction. Proponents also argue that it affords a better chance at creating a smooth contour. Now, I've seen photos of patients who have had the procedure done, and I've taken the courses myself, but right now I'm not convinced that it's that much of an advantage over conventional liposuction. That's because the drawbacks to the procedure outweigh the benefits in my mind. For example, there are larger stab wounds for insertion of the cannulas, which are the tubes that are inserted under the skin to remove the fat. In addition to the tube used to suck out fat, you also need the tube that produces the sound waves to liquefy the fat. The procedure takes longer, which translates to more operating room time, and it costs more than other types of liposuction.

"Ultrasonic liposuction may become a more viable option in the future when its indications and advantages have been more thoroughly worked out. Right now, it's certainly not the best treatment for every patient in every situation. No gadgetry can replace a well-planned, meticulously performed surgery."

Once I was sure that Donna understood the procedure and that her general questions had been answered, we changed the subject and talked about her past medical history and her family history. Donna's medical history was notable for hay fever and an occasional migraine headache. She had been taking Fiorinal for her headaches and had also been taking birth control pills. Because there can be some bleeding with the liposuction procedure, I ordered blood work on her and, happily, the tests all came back normal.

After we finished going over her medical history, I escorted her to the exam room and handed her a gown. I left the room to allow her time to change in privacy. A few minutes later, I knocked at the door and found her sitting in the examination chair waiting patiently.

I asked her to stand in front of the mirror, while I sat down on the stool just to the right of the mirror, near the examination chair. I warned her that this is the hard part: I wanted her to pretend that I wasn't there and talk out loud, as if she were talking to herself, about the areas that she wanted suctioned and the kinds of changes she would like to see. *Clarity is power.* I asked her to be very precise in describing what she wanted to happen.

Donna paused for a while and then walked toward the mirror, sizing herself up. "Right here, to start with," she said as she pointed to her lateral thighs, "this has got to go." She then grabbed two fist-fuls of abdominal wall and added, "My stomach, too." She turned away from the mirror and looked me square in the eye. "That's it. These are the areas I'm most concerned about, my stomach and my thighs."

I understood generally what Donna wanted. The next step was to take some Polaroid pictures. I do this whenever my examination re-quires that the patient be undressed. This way we both have some-thing to evaluate and the patient doesn't have to stand there nude while we discuss the operation. The pictures would help both of us to see exactly what we were talking about and are instrumental in planning the surgery.

At first, Donna balked at the suggestion. "Pictures of this fat?" she said. "I'm not so sure I want that."

I assured her that her face wouldn't be in the photos. Donna stood in front of a blue background that was designed to enhance both the look and the contrast of the pictures. I moved quickly to shorten her ordeal. I took Polaroids in three views—straight on, from the side, and finally from the back. I then handed Donna back her gown. I asked her to get dressed and meet me in the office.

I had already begun to draw on the photographs when Donna en-tered the room. She stared first at the pictures and then at me. She was obviously surprised. I think it's fair to say that a lot of people look in the mirror, but until you take a picture and physically place it in front of them, they can't be critical about what they see. A pic-ture seems to allow them to see their body as not belonging to them. They become a bystander who can give a more honest opinion of what they see.

I pushed the pictures to the center of the table in front of us, and showed her the areas that I thought needed to be addressed.

"My god," Donna interrupted. "That's me? It's worse than I thought."

I reassured her that it wasn't that bad. "Just stay with me," I said. I began with the frontal view, first trimming off the bulges of the lateral thighs. Just above the bulges of the lateral thighs was an indentation. I pointed this out to Donna. This represents the greater trochanter, or hipbone. The muscles attach here and this area can be used to identify the lateral contour of the suctioning. Just above the greater trochanter are the bulges that represent fat deposits in the posterior hips. The bulges below represent fat deposits in the lateral thighs. When I contour the lateral thighs, I think it's important to blend both of these areas into this landmark above and below.

Next I showed Donna that there were areas of her hips and medial knee that also contributed to the contour of her legs.

Then we turned to the lateral view. I asked her to take a good look at her umbilicus, or belly button. The depth of the belly button gives us some idea of where the abdominal wall truly is. That makes it easy to see how much of the abdomen needs to go. With that, I drew a straight line that contoured the protrusion of her abdomen to equal the level of her umbilicus. The upper abdomen, or epigastrium, needs to be addressed, too. I then connected these two areas to show her what the end result would look like when these areas had been contoured to the level of the umbilicus.

After she was comfortable with that, I suggested we take a look at the posterior view. I was quick to point out that this is really a continuation of the frontal view. What I wanted Donna to remember, and what I try to instill in each patient, is that pictures are two-dimensional structures that represent the body, which is three-dimensional. So even though we're drawing straight lines, what we're really talking about is taking off a certain volume, not a specific area that exists in a two-dimensional plane. After I showed her

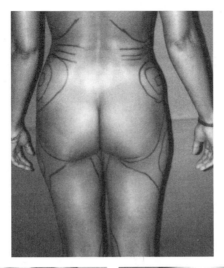

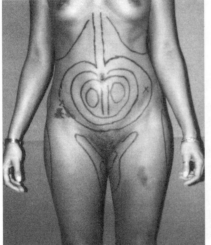

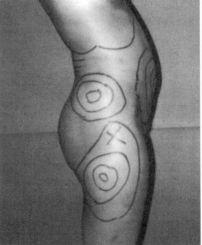

Figure 11: Preoperative markings used in suction-assisted lipectomy (liposuction).

a continuation of the areas to be addressed, I turned to Donna and once again offered some reassurance.

I wanted her to understand that she was a good candidate for liposuction. She was healthy, athletic, and exercised regularly. The bulges that she had weren't generalized fat but isolated pockets. I was confident that her problem areas would respond very well to the procedure.

"So what's next?" Donna asked.

The Procedure

We'd covered almost everything except the procedure itself. I like to get started around 7:30 in the morning, which means I try to have patients arrive at the surgery center at about 6:30 A.M. At this time, the nurses get you signed in, and you meet the anesthesiologist. The anesthesiologist will have probably called you the night before and he will ask you questions that you've already answered, but that's for safety. Bear with him. Everyone is on your side, and I want things to run as smoothly as possible.

I generally show up around 7:00. I meet you in the preoperative holding area, where you and I will really do the surgery. We will mark the areas to be suctioned using concentric circles. It's important that you participate, so that we're sure to address the areas that are of most concern to you. We'll agree on the placement of the stab wounds to insert the cannula. I generally try to put them in areas where they will be hidden, and that includes the gluteal folds, which are just below the buttocks, the navel, and sometimes the groin when we're addressing the medial thighs. If we're also going to do the medial knee, then I put a stab wound in the bend of the knee, the crease that you see on the back side of the leg. After we finish the markings, the surgery is practically done. It's just a matter of physically doing it.

The anesthesiologist then puts in an IV and you are taken to the operating room, where you're gently put to sleep. I normally use general anesthesia for this procedure. It makes for a more pleasant experience, and frankly, I think that's what the patient deserves. I know that there are people who advertise doing this under local at lunchtime, but I don't think that's how it should be done. As far as I'm concerned, that's just a selling tool to get you in the office. The object here is to make a smooth, flat surface using a round cannula. I find that no matter where I make these circles, I end up feathering outside of them to smooth the areas. When I'm doing this under local anesthesia, that means going outside the anesthetized area, which hurts the patient.

My point is, why should the operation hurt? General anesthesia is very safe, and it works better than a local, particularly if we're doing two or three different areas. I can also use less local anesthetic, and the less medicine infused, the safer it is for the patient. Besides, let's face it, with a gentle general anesthesia, you come to the surgery center, go peacefully off to sleep, and wake up when it's all over.

After the anesthesiologist gets you to sleep, the nurses wash the areas to be suctioned and sterile drapes are applied. At this point, you get an intravenous antibiotic and the local anesthetic. The local generally consists of lidocaine, epinephrine, and saline. I do this basically to minimize the amount of bleeding. After allowing enough time for the local to work, we make the stab wounds and inject the tumescent fluid. The tumescent technique is the process of injecting fluid all around the areas to be suctioned. The fluid contains epinephrine, lidocaine, and sometimes some steroids. These agents work together to reduce bleeding and minimize swelling. I give this fluid ten to twenty minutes to work and then begin the procedure.

To do your abdomen and thighs, for instance, we're talking about an hour to an hour and a half of operating time. It could be a little more, it could be a little less. The issue here is not to rush; I take my time and work meticulously. Afterward, we put you in a compression garment, which is really a girdle. The garment will probably get a little stained with blood over the first two days, but I want you to tolerate this and leave everything in place. The stab wounds are left open rather than sewn closed. I've found that if you leave them open, they serve to drain excess fluid and old blood, but most importantly, as they heal they contract down to a little point, leaving a less noticeable scar. When I sew them, you end up with a fine-line scar about 1 cm in length that is more noticeable.

Postoperative Follow-Up

Postoperatively, I'll see you two days after the operation to make certain that everything is OK, and then seven days afterward to make sure that the bruising is minimal and that you are healing well. After three weeks, we'll start you back to your regular activity and increase this over the next three weeks to get you back to normal. So we're really talking about six weeks before you're back to your old self.

Before Donna's consultation was over, we needed to discuss some of the misconceptions about liposuction and some of the problems that can occur with surgery.

Commonly Asked Questions

· **Should I diet before surgery?** Many people wonder if they should try to lose weight before their surgery. The answer is *no*. Liposuction is a body contour procedure, not a weight loss procedure. It makes no sense to starve yourself, especially because lack of nutrition impedes healing. Nor does it make any sense to work out five hours a day if that's not something you already do. You want your weight to be at its normal, steady state. That's important so that the changes that you get during surgery will last. Let's face it, no one starves themselves forever and no one exercises five hours a day forever. If you starve yourself before liposuction and then afterward go back to eating regularly, you set yourself up for failure. It's stupid. You will gain weight under those circumstances.

· *Is liposuction only for younger people?* Doctors used to believe that only people who were young and thin with isolated pockets of fat and good skin turgor were good candidates. Turgor is the ability of the skin to be elastic and to snap back to its original shape or contract around areas where tissue has been removed. We now know that just about everyone can benefit from liposuction. Age is not a deterrent, nor is skin elasticity per se. A great number of older people have demonstrated that their skin can accommodate suctioning. In fact, I've suctioned people who were over seventy years of age.

· *What parts of my body can be contoured by liposuction?* These days, nearly any area of the body can be suctioned with favorable results. This includes the face, arms, neck, back, buttocks and thighs, abdomen, knees, calves, and lower legs.

Complications

Here are some possible complications that are specific to liposuction.

· *Pigment changes.* The bruising that one sees following liposuction represents blood that is out of the vascular (blood vessel) system and trapped under the skin. The body therefore has to reabsorb this blood. As it does, the breakdown product of the blood cells includes a dark pigment that can cause darkening of the skin. Pigmentary changes can be prevented by minimizing bruising. In this regard, the compression garment is your best friend. Wear it religiously and it will work to prevent this problem.

· *Contour irregularities.* Everyone has heard horror stories about people winding up with irregularities in their thighs. These types of contour problems have largely been solved by using smaller cannulas. Now, I know that there are some plastic

surgeons who promote the fact that they're using smaller cannulas as a selling tool. Believe me, it's only marketing. Today
we all use pretty much the same technique and we all use
smaller cannulas. The difference in results has to do with taking
your time and paying attention to detail.

· ***Oversuctioning.*** If too much fat is taken out, it can lead to
skin wrinkling. This can sometimes be corrected by suctioning
adjacent areas, excising skin, fat injections, and time. Some surgeons have even used endomology, or ultrasound, to address this
problem. I think it's fair to say that they all work to a certain de-
gree, but it makes more sense to avoid the problem by doing the
proper preoperative preparation.

When you talk about complications, though, you also have to
mention those problems that can occur with any surgery. They include bleeding with hematoma formation, infection, wound separation, tissue death, injury to nerves, and lung problem including
pulmonary embolism.

The Cost of Liposuction

Finally Donna and I got to the make-or-break issue for a single mom
with law school student loans hanging over her head: the cost of the
procedure. The price of liposuction depends on the number of areas
that are being suctioning. The fixed prices are generally anywhere
from $600 to $1,000 for the anesthesia, and from $1,200 to $1,500
for the operating room, depending on the amount of time the surgeon takes. The price for a major liposuction area like the thighs or
the abdomen is $3,000 with the surgeon generally charging approx-
imately $1,000 for each additional area. In the case of thighs and ab-
domen, we're looking at a total of approximately $5,800. Donna's
surgery, including suctioning her knees, cost a total of $6,300.

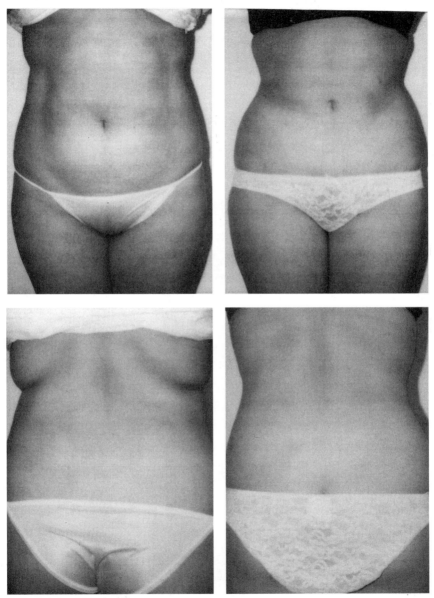

Figure 12: Pre- and postoperative photo of a 31-year-old female with sculpting of the abdomen and flanks (liposuction) to recreate a natural waistline. Of particular note, the excess fat beneath the bra line in the posterior view has been dramatically improved.

Donna called the office with numerous questions over the next few months. Sometimes she would ask technical questions about the surgery, and sometimes she would attempt to renegotiate the price.

Finally, after about four months of trying, she convinced the office staff that she should get her surgery done for a total of $5,000, because that was all she had. To her surprise, and at their convincing, I agreed, and about five months after her initial consultation she underwent the liposuction just in time for her wedding.

As I had pointed out earlier, she was an excellent candidate and her result was fantastic. She spent her honeymoon in Hawaii. And by the way, she passed her bar exam!

11

Mastopexy (Breast Lift)

What Is Breast Ptosis?

BREAST PTOSIS, OR SAGGING, is a common problem for women, especially those who have large breasts or who have had children. There are a number of factors that cause the problem. Gravity is one culprit, especially in large breasts. Sagging is also often the result of pregnancy. During pregnancy, hormones cause the breasts to enlarge. Then postpartum, there's a loss of volume in the upper quadrants when a woman's hormones return to normal. In effect, this leaves the breasts stretched out. When you take a woman in her thirties who has had a few kids and add gravity to the equation, the results can be disastrous. Any time there is an increase in breast volume and then it's taken away, you get sagging. Ptosis can also be a side effect of massive weight loss and can occur during the hormonal changes associated with menopause.

There are different levels of breast ptosis. From a plastic surgery standpoint, the amount of sagging is quantified by the relationship between the level of the nipple and the inframammary fold. This classification system enables plastic surgeons to assess the magnitude of the problem and decide on the most effective therapy.

- *Grade 1 ptosis.* The nipple rests above the level of the inframammary fold. The suprasternal notch to nipple distance is within normal limits, at approximately 21 cm. There is some sagging of the lower portion of the breast itself, but the major deformity is the result of loss of volume in the upper quadrant. In a sense, the upper part of the breast is flat. So even though the substance of the breast itself has not fallen significantly below prepregnancy level, the net effect is that the breast sags because of loss of projection and tissue in the upper quadrant.

· *Grade 2 ptosis.* The nipple falls below the inframammary fold but still remains above the lowest contour of the breast. This presents a situation in which the suprasternal notch to nipple distance has increased to greater than 21–22 cm, usually around 24 cm. The net effect is the appearance of a massive loss of tissue and breast projection.

· *Grade 3 ptosis.* The nipple is the lowest contour of the breast and extends both below the lowest contour of the breast itself and below the inframammary fold.

· *Pseudo-ptosis.* This condition is characterized by a loose flat breast in which the nipple is above the inframammary fold. The suprasternal notch to nipple distance remains the same as in the prepregnancy state, yet massive loss of volume in the upper quadrant postpartum gives the illusion of breast sagging.

Ptosis Solutions

Once we know the level of the nipple from the suprasternal notch, the nipple's relation to the inframammary fold, and the amount of excess skin in the upper quadrant, the surgeon can decide what is the best solution for the problem.

THE PSEUDO-PTOSIS SOLUTION

The best solution for this situation is usually augmentation mammoplasty. Again, the nipple has not descended, and therefore does not need to be raised. There is no need to remove skin. The major problem in this case is lack of volume in the upper quadrants bilaterally. Augmentation mammoplasty solves this problem with the minimum amount of trauma to the patient and the minimum amount of scarring. The result is a full and voluptuous breast that is in tune with the patient's body size and available skin envelope.

THE GRADE 1 PTOSIS SOLUTION
Again, the best solution for this situation is usually augmentation mammoplasty. The nipple is at the level of the inframammary fold. This condition may be compromised by skin that is elastotic (i.e. lost its ability to return to initial shape) and therefore has lost a great deal of its turgor. Therefore, its important to make sure the skin envelope is not so loose that the weight of the implants—and gravity—causes further sagging. In this situation, a small amount of skin around the nipple can be removed to raise the breast. This procedure, called the peri-areolar round block technique, or Bennelli lift, works very well for women with a minimum amount of sagging. The breast lift is accomplished by excising a doughnut of skin around the areola. The nipple is then raised to an appropriate level. The scar produced is barely noticeable because it's around the areolar complex at the junction where the dark areolar skin joins the lighter skin of the breast. A nonabsorbable suture is woven around the nipple areolar complex and its diameter is fixed by tying the suture. This supports some of the tension on the areolar complex from the might of the implant, and therefore helps preserve the shape and size of the areolar complex. Without this peri-areolar suture, the nipple areolar complex can become enlarged or distorted postoperatively. Other potential problems with this procedure include the possibility of developing a hypertrophic scar around the nipple areolar complex, and some flattening of the breast contour.

GRADE 2 AND GRADE 3 PTOSIS SOLUTION

In this situation, the surgeon must estimate the amount of skin that needs to be removed, and some skin does in fact need to be removed. This is accomplished using the Wise pattern, a technique that's also used in breast reductions. What it does is allow the surgeon to raise the nipple areolar complex to the appropriate level and at the same time remove excess skin. The surplus skin is the result of stretching of the lower quadrants of the breast. The downside to this procedure is the inverted T-shaped scar, the same type you get with a breast reduction. The upside is that the breast can often be lifted and the projection of the breast returned without the placement of an implant. If an implant is required to obtain the desired look, it must be placed prior to reducing the skin envelope so that an adequate amount of skin remains to accommodate the implant.

Perking Up Pamela

When Pamela came to my office, she was tired of feeling miserable about her sagging breasts. Although she had a beautiful smile, her eyes looked tired and her demeanor was somewhat as if she had been beaten down. Pamela was thirty-eight years old and in the middle of a divorce. Nevertheless, she seemed fairly healthy psychologically. She'd finally resolved that the divorce was really best for everyone involved. She was ready to get on with her life. Pamela said she'd been considering a breast lift for the last three years; now she was ready to do it. She had been a C cup prior to having children, but she'd lost volume in her breasts and was distraught about what she described as "massive sagging."

She began our consultation quite bluntly. "I need to talk to you about two things, she said, "my breasts. They sag, and after I had my children, they simply dropped down to my waist. I can't stand it.

I've lost a lot of size. I was a C cup before I had kids. Now I'm an A. I'm not sure I want them bigger, but I certainly want them up."

Our initial consultation began by examining the causes of ptosis, or drooping. I explained that her problem was probably due to a combination of gravity, loss of skin elasticity, atrophy of the breasts' fatty layer due to removal of the pregnancy hormones after delivery, and to some extent heredity or genetics.

In her case, I was concerned that there were a great number of stretch marks in the upper quadrants of her breasts. This suggested to me that a breast implant alone would only complicate the drooping after a few months, causing even more sagging than she had now. The major problem in this particular circumstance is the loss of turgor, or elasticity of the skin, due to the stretch marks. Stretch marks are scars in which the underlying dermal layers of skin have been torn and subsequently heal. This process damages the skin and makes the tissue less elastic.

Pamela's suprasternal notch to nipple distance was 25 cm on the right and 24.5 cm on the left. In my opinion, elevating her breasts to a level of 21 to 22 cm would result in more than enough breast volume for her body size. I suggested a mastopexy, or breast lift, for her rather than implants. I felt that if we got her breasts up and excised some of the tissue, they would be perky enough to satisfy her.

I was afraid she would object to the scarring associated with a breast lift, rather than an augmentation mammoplasty. But she said right away that the scars themselves would not be an issue for her. Her concern was just getting her breasts off her stomach. She figured that the scars would be covered by a bra or swimsuit.

I told her that once the breasts had been elevated to the appropriate level, we could add an implant at a later date if she was not satisfied with the volume. It was important to point out also that this did not represent the same situation as trying to place an implant immediately, at the time of skin resection. By delaying the procedure, the skin has time to heal and to establish adequate blood flow. At six months to a year later, the threat to the skin through loss of adequate blood flow and nutrition is less. Also, the skin would have had time to soften the scars, so the tissue would be more pliable. However, she would have to wait at least six months after the first procedure before we could add the implant. Though she was not completely happy about the possibility of having to wait so long and have two surgeries, she understood that this was the safest, most effective way to achieve the most perfect results in her situation.

Pamela had a history of stomach ulcers, but at the time of our consultation she was not on any medication, nor had she had any recent stomach problems. Her blood counts were perfect; in fact, they were higher than expected. Generally, women in this age group who are still experiencing menses have hemoglobin and hematocrit counts that are a bit low. The hemoglobin refers to the amount of iron in the blood, while the hematocrit is a ratio of the blood cell volume of cells to the fluid component of blood.

The Mastopexy Procedure

A mastopexy is similar to a breast reduction procedure. The difference is that only skin is removed, not breast tissue. I started telling Pamela what she could expect:

On the night before surgery, I said, you'll get a call from the anesthesiologist. He'll go over your medical history and ask a lot of the same questions that I asked you today. On the morning of the procedure, you should arrive at the surgery center one hour prior to the surgery. At this point, you and I will do the Wise pattern markings in the preoperative holding area. Those are exactly the markings that one would perform if doing a breast reduction. The Wise pattern is designed to show the surgeon where to remove skin and/or breast tissue when attempting to lift the breast from a sagging position to a more prominent and normal "perky" position. After this is done and we agree upon the nipple placement, we'll identify the amount of skin to be excised from the lower portion of the breasts. When this skin is removed, the result will be a lift in the breast contour.

Then we move to the operating room, where you are placed on your back and gently put to sleep by the anesthesiologist. The nurses wash your chest, arms, abdomen, and breasts with a Betadine soap solution. Then they paint your chest with a Betadine paint solution to kill all the bacteria on the skin in this area. We use sterile drapes to partition off the chest area and exclude the rest of your body from the operative field. You'll be given intravenous antibiotics.

We begin the procedure by excising the skin in the areas that we marked in the preoperative holding area. Your breasts are then fashioned into a conical shape, and the incision lines are closed using a subcuticular closure. That means I'll use dissolvable sutures that are placed underneath the skin. This helps minimize the amount of scarring and does away with the problem of suture marks on the skin itself.

Postoperative Care

After the procedure, you are taken from the operating room to the recovery room, where you are monitored until you are completely awake. You'll have a bulky dressing around your breasts that consists of Steri-strips, which are thin tapes to hold the skin edges together and lend support to the skin closure. This in turn is covered with gauze sponges, and the whole area is wrapped with six-inch Ace wraps for comfort. You'll remain at the surgical center until you're completely awake, able to urinate, and can swallow liquids. Then you're discharged and allowed to leave with the person who is driving you home.

Before you leave, I'll give you prescriptions for approximately five days of pain medicine and five days of antibiotics if you don't already have them. Then I'll see you two days after the procedure to make sure that everything is healing well. I like to leave the dressing on for forty-eight hours because theoretically it was placed on in a sterile condition and will stay that way until it is disturbed. By waiting forty-eight hours before changing your bandages, the wound has time to seal and the likelihood of bacteria contamination is minimized. I see you again approximately one week after the operation to remove any sutures or Steri-strips. Following this visit, you can wash your breasts and the incision line gently with soap and water and apply Neosporin or Bacitracin ointment to the incision line at least twice a day. At three weeks postoperatively, you can start back to your regular activities. We'll see each other again approximately two months after the procedure and six months after the procedure, to take any postoperative photos.

The Cost Of Mastopexy

The breast mastopexy procedure takes approximately three hours, which translates into a $1,600 fee for the surgical facility. The anesthesia is another $650 to $1,000. The surgeon's fee can run anywhere from $5,000 to $6,000, making the total approximately $8,250. This includes any supplies and postoperative visits you may require.

The breast lift, or mastopexy, is a procedure that makes the patients feel incredibly good about themselves. Psychologically, it can go a long way toward reestablishing a woman's self-esteem. I had a feeling that Pamela would benefit both physically and mentally from this surgery.

I love it when a successful surgery makes my patients look and feel better. But I've learned to evaluate the demeanor of patients whose psychological profile does not change, even when they get the surgical results they hoped for. They *still* feel bad about themselves.

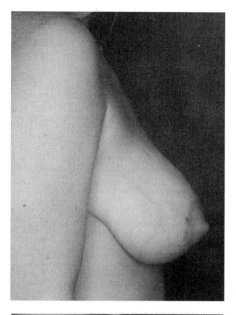

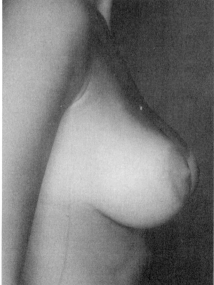

Figure 13: Mastopexy (Breast Lift). This 41-year-old female underwent a breast lift procedure. Although the scars are similar to that
of a breast reduction, no breast tissue is removed. Only the excess
skin—which results in sagging of the breast—is excised. In some
cases a lift can be obtained via augmentation.

In a sense, it comes down to how one chooses to look at things. I know from seeing these patients' lack of progress that I always want to be able to see the good side of a situation. In fact, I've come to realize that looking on the bright side can take you further in life than a Harvard education.

I wanted to share this philosophy with Pamela because I knew she was going through a tough spot in her own life. Certainly, divorce is psychologically challenging, even when it's the right thing to do. I told her I believed that 90 percent of what's going on in our lives is good, and about 10 percent is not so good. Many of us have a tendency to focus on the bad 10 percent instead of the 90 percent that's good. Focusing on the good 90 percent is the key to being happy and successful.

I hugged her and told her that things would be all right. I couldn't help myself. We'd had such a good talk that I felt like she was a close friend or my daughter. I knew this strong woman was going to come out on top.

Pamela went through the surgery with flying colors. The surgery gave her the lift she needed, and she was able to get through her divorce with as little pain as one could expect. I know she decided to take a healthy look at what she was going through, even though on her postoperative visits she seemed more intellectual about what she was going through rather than dealing with what she felt. I guess that's what she needed at the time.

She was clear, though, that she wasn't ready to start dating, and by her last postoperative visit at six months, she hadn't. I hope she does soon, because I'm sure she'll make someone very happy.

12

Abdominoplasty (Tummy Tuck)

THE ABDOMEN IS OFTEN a problem area for women of color in their thirties. When a patient is considering rejuvenative surgery in this region, the first thing we discuss is her reproductive history. Knowing if she's had children helps me to identify what her needs will be. That is, it gives me an idea of whether the best procedure will be simple liposuction or a complete abdominoplasty, known as a tummy tuck. This discussion also gives us a chance to address any initial concerns and develop a rapport before the physical examination, which goes a long way toward making a patient feel comfortable. Getting undressed in front of a stranger isn't easy. Most of my patients are shy and embarrassed—especially if they feel they've let their abdomen get out of control. I try to reassure them that I'm not here to judge them; I'm here to help solve their problem and make them feel good about themselves again.

How to Tell if Your Abdomen Needs Liposuction or a Tummy Tuck

The way to tell if you need liposuction or an abdominoplasty is based on whether you have an excess of subcutaneous fat (known as lipodystrophy), or whether you have an excess of fat *and* skin (known as dermatolipodystrophy). Excess fat can usually be remedied by liposuction; getting rid of both excess fat and skin requires a tummy tuck.

Many women who've had children need the tummy tuck rather than liposuction. This has to do with what happens to the abdomen during pregnancy. Let's start by discussing the layers of the abdominal wall, which include skin, subcutaneous fat, fascia, which is the fibrous covering of the muscle, then the muscle. Deep to the muscle is a flimsy layer of tissue called the peritoneum, which is a sac that contains the intra-abdominal cavity and its contents, the stomach organs.

In an individual who has had children, the uterus, which sits in the intra-abdominal cavity, expands to accommodate the enlarging fetus. As a result, the abdominal wall is stretched, including all of the aforementioned layers. The skin, the fat, and the muscle and peritoneal layers are very elastic and have the ability to stretch and return to their normal state without much problem (although if the stretching is too fast, stretch marks can form in the skin, causing it to sag). The fascia, however, which is fibrous in nature, does not always return to its original state. This accounts for the protrusion of the lower abdomen that is seen postpartum even in thin women. What has happened is that the sac that is one's belly has become larger. This is complicated by the fact that the bowels and other intra-abdominal contents move into this new larger space. A person with this problem requires an abdominoplasty. All the liposuction and all the sit-ups in the world aren't going to correct the fact that the entire abdominal cavity has become larger and, more important, looser.

If stretching of the abdomen due to a pregnancy occurs too fast, the result is stretch marks. Stretch marks are scars underneath the skin. This scar has replaced the elastic tissue and that is why in the areas of stretch marks, the skin sags. It is devoid of elastic tissue. This problem also needs to be addressed with abdominoplasty.

In someone who has not had children, chances are that the abdominal layers have not been stretched and the excess abdomen represents an increase in the size of the subcutaneous fatty layer. This type of problem responds very well to liposuction.

Diane: Upset About her Stomach

Diane came to see me with her husband in tow. Despite fifteen years of marriage and five kids, it was obvious that they shared the type of love that many of us only experience as teenagers. Their relationship was mature and had weathered the rigors of everyday life, but it was clearly passionate. Diane's husband was quiet and friendly, while she was very outgoing with a tremendously inviting smile. That smile was simply infectious. She was loud, too, and I liked that. Her personality made me feel like I was with my relatives.

At thirty-eight, Diane was thick and athletic, but you couldn't really call her fat. She was thick through the hips, buttocks, and thighs, but soft and petite up top. Her concern was her belly. Five children had left her with a huge pouch that she couldn't get rid of with exercise. She had grown self-conscious, and the clothes that she wore were indicative of that. Diane was dressed in black stretch pants with sneakers. Her choice of tops, though, was the giveaway. It was large—very large—with long sleeves, and hung low around her hips to cover her stomach and rear without clinging to either one.

Diane had been trying to lose weight, but she was not on any medications. She did complain that she bruised easily, but there were no bruises on her. She did not take aspirin on a regular basis. Of her five pregnancies, the last two had been delivered by Cesarean section. Generally, her past medical history was very good.

Diane opted to conduct her physical exam without her husband present. This is often the case, as people just feel more comfortable with fewer people looking at them. Her abdomen was very protuberant, with stretch marks beginning almost at the level of her ribs and extending down her pubis. Her belly button was pushed out like a softball, and the integrity of the midline of her abdomen was completely gone. There was no support of her midline abdomen, and this clearly explained the protuberance of her belly. In addition to having dermatolipodystrophy of the abdomen with a diastasis recti, or separation of the rectus muscles, she also had a large ventral hernia. The hernia, which is a protrusion of the intra-abdominal contents as a result of a weakening or defect in the abdominal wall, was her major problem. No wonder exercise wasn't working for her. No wonder she was frustrated.

As Diane got dressed privately in the exam room, her husband pulled me aside. He wanted me to understand how important this procedure was to both him and Diane. Diane's figure had made her so depressed that her personality had changed. I reassured him that we could solve the problem. When Diane was dressed, we returned to the office, where we sat down to discuss what would be the best plan for her.

I said that Diane needed an abdominoplasty. She was a perfect candidate for a tummy tuck, which would alleviate the bulging in her abdomen caused by too much skin and fat. But she also needed to have her ventral hernia repaired. I suggested that she go to see her primary medical doctor, because her insurance would probably pay for some of the surgery. She needed her primary care physician to document the problem for insurance purposes, but I reassured her that I would do the surgery. Her large ventral hernia was clearly caused by her pregnancies and the previous Caesarian sections. I wanted her to understand the root of her problem in the hopes that she would no longer blame herself.

Next I told Diane and her husband about the procedure itself. The purpose of the abdominoplasty is to restore a prepregnancy contour to the anterior abdominal wall.

I asked Diane to bring her skimpiest underwear or bathing suit with her to the surgical center. The reason for this is that I want to place the incision within the panty line of this garment so that once its on, no one can see the incision. If you're going to have a tummy tuck, you're going to have a scar, period. The question is to what extent. Almost any doctor can cut off the excess skin, but one of the reasons you go to a plastic surgeon is because you want your scarring to be minimized to accommodate your lifestyle.

I explained that while you're in preop, I mark the incision line within the contour of your panties or bathing suit. Then you sit down and talk with the anesthesiologist, who will go over your medical history and discuss the process of anesthesia with you. Next you are taken to the operating room, where an intravenous line will be put in your arm to give you fluids and medications. You are placed on your back on the operating room table. Care is taken to position you so that your hip area is at a level where the bed can be folded. This allows us to move the bed in order to flex your body. We do this to maximize the amount of excess skin that can be taken out and still allow for an adequate closure of the incisions. Then the nurses wash your body from your knees to your shoulders with a Betadine soap solution. They'll also paint your body with an antibacterial Betadine solution. After this is complete, the abdomen is isolated from the rest of your body with sterile drapes to keep the operative field clean.

After you've been gently put to sleep, I make the incision in the proposed site using a small scalpel, and then use electrocautery to cut down through the subcutaneous tissue to the level of the muscle fascia. [Electrocautery is the use of an instrument that emits a small amount of electricity to seal up blood vessels as it cuts through them. This is done to minimize bleeding.] Once I'm down to the level of the muscle fascia, I'll raise a flap of skin and subcutaneous tissue up to the level of the belly button. The belly button is then circumscribed and cut out, allowing it to remain in its normal location. I then continue to raise the flap of skin and subcutaneous tissue up to the level of the costal arch, which is the lower level of the ribs. What we end up with is a sheet of skin and fat that extends from your pubis to your rib cage.

After the flap is raised, I tighten the fascia underneath with sutures. This is done by using a pen and marking an ellipse on your abdomen that extends from the middle of the rib cage, or xiphoid, which is the bottom tip of your chest bone or sternum, down to the area of the pubis. The belly button is the center of this ellipse. The fascia is then sewn in from the sides to tighten your waist and the anterior abdominal wall. This is done in two layers to reinforce the suturing. Then, as I noted earlier, we flex the bed at the hips to maximize the amount of skin that can be removed. The skin is then stretched, inset, and trimmed appropriately. I'll close the midsection of the incision line using dissolvable sutures to approximate the deep tissues. A running subcuticular suture is used to close the skin. Next, through the open lateral aspect of the wound, I locate the belly button, make an incision in the skin directly above the belly button, pull it through the incision, inset it, and sew it. After that is complete, drains will be placed in the lateral aspect of the wounds.

Most people have a great deal of concern about the drains, but they are your best friends. Drains are essentially tubes that prevent fluid from collecting in the layers between the skin and fat flap and the muscle fascia layer. If you think about it, this layer needs to stick down in order to heal; if fluid accumulates, it can't do that. The drains may stay in from five to seven days or longer. How long they stay in has nothing to do with how you're doing, or the length of time it will take to heal. Some people simply drain more fluid than others. The drains are just there to protect you. They will be removed when the drainage is minimal.

Once the drains have been placed, we will close the lateral aspect of the incision and then place the drains to self-suction. The self-suction mechanisms are plastic balls that attach to the ends of the drains.

These produce suction when they're squeezed flat, and a cap is placed on while the container is collapsed. The nurses will teach you how to empty and reconnect these drains so that you can do this at home.

While you're still asleep, you will be placed onto another flexed bed so you can be moved to the recovery room. The position of the bed ensures that there is no tension on your abdominal closure. You will then be gently awakened from sleep and wheeled to the recovery room. Here you'll be given fluids until you are fully awake. You may or may not have a catheter in your bladder to drain urine. This will be taken out prior to your discharge from the surgical center.

The Postoperative Period

The postoperative period begins once you are discharged from the operating room. You will have five to seven days of pain medication and five days of antibiotics to take orally. You'll feel some tightness in your abdominal area, and you will be unable to stand up straight because of the skin excision. You may feel as if you will pull your sutures apart, but that won't happen. It will, however, take you a few days to go from the bent-over, flexed position to being completely upright.

On the first day, I want you to get out of bed and walk around your house with assistance. You will not be able to stand up straight, but the pulling and tightness that you feel are normal, and there is no chance of separating the wound. I will see you in the office on postoperative day two. We will take the dressing down, we examine the drains to make sure that they are functioning properly, and we change the dressing. In some cases, I leave the wound open so you can wash the incision line two to three times a day with soap and water. Controlling the drains and taking care of the incision line is something that you can do at home. Therefore, I won't see you again for approximately five days.

On day seven I'll see you again. At this time, we remove all sutures and drains. I ask that you continue to take it easy over the next two weeks. By this point you will be able to walk without assistance, and I suggest that you do so as much as you can tolerate. At three weeks postoperatively, you'll start back to your regular activities. It will take about three more weeks before you're back to normal. For example, if you were accustomed to running three miles a day, I would suggest during this first week of regular activity that you run one mile, and during the second week you run two miles. Therefore, by the third week—that is, six weeks after surgery—you'll be back to your three-mile run. I will see you again at approximately three months to take postoperative photographs.

Possible Complications

As with any surgery, there are certain complications associated with this procedure to be aware of.

- **Wound separation.** Separation of the wound can occur if healing does not take place due to inadequate blood flow. If there is too much tension on the flap, it results in decreasing the amount of blood flow into the flap, much like when one applies pressure to a finger. The wound separation occurs at the time of suture removal. Though a problem at the time, these wounds heal very well secondarily by allowing them to close on their own and do not necessarily require further surgery. This is a technical error and requires adequate planning by the surgeon in order to avoid it.
- *Separation of the umbilicus from its placement.* This is also due to tension and subsequent loss of adequate blood flow. It represents too much pulling on the stalk of the belly button as a result of placing it too high or too low on the flap.

· *Seroma formation.* A seroma is a collection of fluid, which is generally straw-colored, under the skin flap. This prevents the flap from sealing down. In order to remedy the problem, the wound must be drained over four to six weeks. This is accomplished by having you come to the office once or twice a week so that we can insert a needle into the seroma to drain it. This complication can usually be avoided by leaving the drains in longer and by being sure that you have stopped draining before they are removed. This is why I tell people that the drains are their friends.

There are other complications that are possible with any surgery. These include bleeding and infection. These are avoided by good surgical technique and paying attention to detail.

The Cost of Abdominoplasty

An abdominal dermatolipectomy, or tummy tuck, requires approximately three hours in the operating room. That means the facility cost for this procedure is $1,600. The anesthesia cost is $650. The surgery itself is $6,500, making a total of $8,750.

However, as Diane and her husband can attest, it is money well spent. After the operation, Diane was a new woman. She felt better about herself and became even more outgoing. Her husband felt like he had his wife back again, after years of depression. They went to Hawaii to celebrate. Diane was so comfortable in her bathing suit that her husband couldn't get her away from the pool. I was thrilled for them.

I was also thrilled to have fixed her hernia. This was done at the same time as her tummy tuck, and from Diane's perspective there was only one operation and she had her stomach back. I took pictures

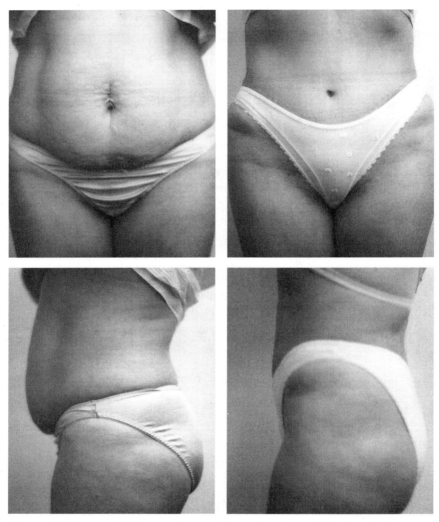

Figure 14: Tummy tuck. Preop and postop photos of a 38-year-old female with diastases recti and redundant abdominal skin.

of her hernia during the operation and noted that in my operative note. For billing purposes, I knew the insurance company would require some documentation before paying for the surgery. To my surprise, they did so without a lot of hassle.

Part Four

The Forties

One of the greatest frustrations that comes with being a physician is knowing that so many diseases and so many medical problems or annoyances could be avoided by taking the right steps to prevent them. Most people never think about a disease or problem until it effects them. Then it is often too late to do anything about it This is true with lung disease, it's true with heart disease, and it's true with aging.

The forties can be either a curse or a blessing. Psychologically, this is a time when you can step forward with confidence as a woman. If you are comfortable with who you are and the choices you've made, you radiate power that is unmistakably real and feminine. On the other hand, if you feel you've made the wrong decisions and relinquished control of your life to others, it can be a period characterized by self-doubt and loneliness. Physically, this is the time when you find out if you've made the right choices to ensure that you age gracefully.

13

Brow Lift/Blepharoplasty (Eyes)

ONE POPULAR MISCONCEPTION IS that people of color show their age less than white people. It is generally held that the signs of facial aging—fine wrinkling, jowling of the jaws, and the sagging of the neck referred to as the turkey gobbler defect—are the bane of Caucasians. The truth, as usual, is more complicated. In general, people of color do tend to show the signs of aging more slowly than whites. But we also age differently, especially in our faces. People of color age more in the brow and eyes, while whites age more in the lower face.

For people of color, the eyes are usually the first part of the face to show the telltale signs of aging. There are a number of factors that contribute to the tired, puffy look that fortysomething women face in the mirror.

- *Fine lines.* This skin becomes less elastic as we age. Often, fine lines around the eyes are the first evidence of this trend.
- *Under-eye bags.* This is a common complaint of patients in their forties. There are a great number of causes of baggy eyes. A loss of elasticity in the skin and the underlying structures has a lot to do with it. The fatty layer surrounding the eye pushes its way out through these structures to form the puffiness that we see in both the upper and lower lids. The periodic swelling that you see in the morning may be associated with the menstrual cycle. It can also be caused by hormonal imbalance, kidney disease, thyroid disease, heart disease, and even alcohol abuse.

- **Droopy brow.** In many cases, the problem of tired-looking eyes isn't localized to the eye area. The brow or forehead drops because of aging, reduced elasticity of the skin, thinning of the subcutaneous fat layer, and in older individuals actual thinning of the skull. All of these conditions contribute to the lateral hooding of the eyes, that droop of the upper eyelid that overhangs the outside of the eye.

- **Muscles.** The muscles of the face also cause changes in the eye area with age. Covering the entire forehead are the paired frontalis muscles that elevate the eyebrows. These muscles are responsible for the transverse forehead lines that occur with aging. In the midline at the root of the nose are the corrugator muscles and the procerus muscle. Their action pulls down the brow, resulting in an angry appearance. The wrinkles that you see at the root of the nose are the result of these muscle actions.

Taken all together, one can see how the combination of a drooping brow, fine wrinkling around the eyes, puffiness, and excess skin all contribute to a look of tiredness.

The eye and brow area is where we focus our attention when we're having a conversation with another person. It is also where we focus when we look at ourselves in the mirror. It's a very visible and important element of our appearance. Yet to some extent, the brow, a major component of this problem, is overlooked in plastic surgery literature.

One reason for this may be that it is difficult to sell a browlift procedure. It involves more extensive surgery than just the eyes. Another reason may be that surgeons don't address the issue because they aren't sure of how to educate patients about the problem. When people come into the office, they're usually focused on their eyes. It is difficult to interrupt their thought pattern and get them to consider other solutions. The idea of a bigger, more extensive surgery is a significant deterrent. But lets face it, the goal is to satisfy patients. And the best way to do that is to solve their problem.

Opening Marie's Eyes

A very pretty forty-two-year-old woman named Marie arrived at my office complaining of puffy, tired eyes. Like many women of color, her first indication of aging was looking in the mirror in the morning after a wonderful night's sleep and noticing that her eyes still looked tired. Marie, however, was beautiful. She was tall and elegant, and the way she dressed screamed confidence. She was wearing a long flowered skirt that gently draped about her hips and legs. Underneath she had on ornate cowboy boots. She wore a peach crew neck sweater and a darker brown sweater tied around her shoulders. Her sunglasses were stylish and very dark. But the icing on the cake, the accessory that set her apart, was her hat. In a way, it was a cowboy hat, but not really. The hat was cloth and around the brim was a snakeskin band. The brim was turned way down in the front and back, covering both her eyes and her dark hair, which was in a ponytail.

Marie was certainly an elegant black woman; she was also very "Beverly Hills." She made her living as a successful screenwriter. There was an air about her that said "I'm in control." She flopped down in the chair in my office and in an exasperated tone said, "It's my eyes. I've got to do something about my eyes."

I asked her what she thought was wrong with her eyes. We both leaned back in our chairs. I examined Marie's face.

"It's really hard to explain," she said. "They look tired, you know, like I'm sleepy. But that doesn't really say it all. Sometimes, but not all the time, my eyes just look puffy or swollen. Also, I'm starting to get some wrinkling around them." She paused for a while and then said, "But I guess that's to be expected."

I told her that the eye area is very complicated and it's difficult to be precise when talking about it. That's partly because the problem isn't always localized to the eyes. Then I said I wanted to do a little experiment. I walked around the table to Marie and gave her a hand-held mirror. I asked her to look in the mirror and focus on her upper eyelids. As Marie stared into the mirror, I placed my thumb on her eyelid and pulled her upper lid upward. I asked if she could see the excess skin of the upper eyelid.

"Sure," she said. "That's what the problem is."

I said that this represented the excess skin in the upper eyelid. However, this was not the whole problem. I relaxed my hold on her upper eyelid skin and then placed my thumb just above her eyebrow and lifted the skin at this level. The loss of redundancy of skin in the upper eyelid was considerable. I then made another attempt to pull out the fold of the skin of the upper eyelid. I asked if she saw how much less skin there was to her upper eyelid now.

Marie nodded.

I explained that the puffiness and elastosis around the eye are only part of the picture. The brow or forehead also drops as we age. Certainly we see the results of this drooping most clearly in the skin around the eyes, but to fix it correctly, we have to go to the root of the problem.

I pointed out the area just outside her eyes, where the excess skin formed a hood over her eyelid. In some people, this gets so bad that they don't have any peripheral vision. Add to this the wrinkling of the forehead due to muscle action, and you've got a complicated problem. It is certainly not just the eyes.

"Okay," Marie interrupted, "but what do we do for me? What's best for me in my situation?"

Usually I'm a surgeon who advocates that less is better, but I also believe that you should have the most appropriate and effective procedure. In Marie's case, I recommended a browlift.

I'm a big advocate of this procedure for women of color because, as I said, this is where we show our age. Our aging is in the eyes and the brow, and this procedure is the best way to combat it. Removing skin from the eyelids isn't usually enough. We also need to get the brow back to its original level. Then the eyelid surgery requires less resection of skin.

It's easy to sell eyelid surgery because people come in wanting it and they see it as a minimal surgery. However, if the problem is brow ptosis and not just the eyelid skin, they get the wrong operation and postoperatively they still have that tired look in their eyes. What generally happens is that patients feel that they didn't get what they paid for and they're unhappy with the results. The surgeon then tries to make a correction and he makes one of two mistakes. He either lifts the brow secondarily and as a result of the previous skin resection of the eyelid, there isn't enough eyelid skin. When this happens, the eyes don't shut, which is an absolute disaster. Or he takes out more skin on the lateral lid and extends the scar unnecessarily onto the temporal area of the face next to the eyelids. Having the right surgery done in the first place is the best way to address these potential complications.

"Wow," Marie said. "I see your point. I really hadn't thought that much about it. I just thought that this tired look was all my eyes. I figured if I got my eyes done, it would all be over."

Next we turned our attention to Marie's lower eyelids. I leaned over to examine Marie's face carefully. I asked her to look straight at me. Then I had her keep her head level and raise only her eyes to look up at the ceiling. This maneuver helps me to get a good look at the fat in the lower lids. Women of color have three special concerns about their lower lids: puffiness, which is caused by a herniation of fat; wrinkles, which are the result of excess skin, sun damage, and muscle action; and hyperpigmentation, which may be caused by inflammation or sun damage. Marie had an excess of both fat and skin, but no hyperpigmentation.

"Okay," Marie said confidently, "that's fine, but tell me exactly what you think I should do, or what you think your plan should be."

I explained that there are two procedures to address the lower lids:

- *The transconjunctival blepharoplasty.* This is done without making an incision in the outside of the skin. This procedure is designed for those people who only have an excess of fat. No skin is removed, so there is no resultant scar on the outside. Simply removing the fat solves the problem. The procedure is accomplished through an incision in the gutter of the eyelid. The gutter is the recess between the skin and the eyeball. The fat is removed from the back of the lid.
- *The standard blepharoplasty.* For patients with an excess of both skin and fat, like Marie, the solution requires both to be excised. The scar, however, is minimal and well hidden. It's placed directly under the eyelashes.

The Browlift

It makes sense to talk about the browlift first because the amount of upper lid skin that we'll excise is determined by the level of the brow. There are two different incisions that we can use, depending on your needs. There is the standard coronal incision that is placed posteriorly in the scalp. The scar is hidden in the hair by placing it 5 to 7 cm behind the hairline. The other is the anterior hairline incision, which is placed at the junction of the forehead and the hair. Both work equally well in women, though the coronal is usually not the best for men because of the possibility of balding. If the hairline recedes, the scar becomes visible. I decide which type of incision to use on my female patients by measuring the length of their forehead. If the distance is greater than 5 cm, I use an anterior hairline incision. If it's less than 5 cm, I use the coronal incision. In other words, the anterior hairline incision shortens the forehead and the coronal incision lengthens it.

In Marie's case, there were a couple of factors to consider. The base of her nose was fine; that is, there was no redundancy of skin, nor were there any wrinkles. As a result, I could avoid an incision in the midline of the brow and just address the lateral hooding of the eye. This is what I mean by less is more, or rather better. I suggested using what we call a bitemporal incision. This incision is placed directly over the lateral aspect of the eye, and the skin is removed at the junction of the hairline with the forehead. This would specifically address Marie's problem of lateral hooding with the least amount of trauma.

Marie then interrupted, "Will people be able to see the scar?"

Not really, I assured her. The incision is in the hair-bearing scalp. Keep in mind, though, that hair doesn't grow where there is a scar. With the anterior hairline incision, the scar is visible when the hair is pulled back. In people who wear bangs, this is not a problem. The coronal incision, however, if it is wide, can look like a part in the hair across the top of the forehead. I try to avoid this complication by zigzagging the incision through the scalp. A zigzag scar is harder to see than a straight-line scar.

Now that we'd figured out what would work best for Marie, I explained the surgery itself. Before the surgery, in the preoperative area, I mark the line of the incision. All the wrinkles in the forehead will be identified and marked. This helps in locating the problem areas during the procedure. I can use either a general or a local anesthesia with sedation. Within reason, I try to consider the patient's preference. If I'm only going to do your forehead, local anesthesia with sedation is reasonable. If we do both the forehead and the eyes, I prefer general anesthesia.

"Can I use local?" she asked. "I'd feel a lot more comfortable. You read all the stories in the papers. I'm just not sure I want to be asleep."

I knew that she was referring to people having problems with anesthesia. Such stories often get reported in the news. What doesn't get reported are the accurate statistics. About ten years ago, the death rate associated with anesthesia was one in 10,000 cases. Today, with better anesthetic techniques, the incidence is estimated at one in 400,000 for all kinds of surgery and much less for those individuals getting cosmetic surgery. I reassured Marie that the anesthesia is quite safe and that I was comfortable in her case using either a local or a general. They both will do the job equally well. I warned her, though, that it can be uncomfortable to have a surgeon working around your eyes. The injections can be painful, and sometimes it takes several to get adequate anesthesia. I want my patients to have a good experience—without pain—so I often recommend general anesthesia. However, if it doesn't bother you to have me working around your eyes, then local is the way to go.

Whether you're asleep or not, I'll inject lidocaine with epinephrine into the surgical field to reduce bleeding. Your face is then washed with a Phisohex soap solution and painted with Betadine. I also use Betadine in your hair, since the temporal incision is in the hairline. This is washed out right after the procedure.

The flesh covering your scalp and forehead has five layers. In order, there is skin; subcutaneous tissue; the aponeurosis, which is a fibrous tissue continuous with the frontalis muscle; the loose areolar tissue; and the periosteum, which is the covering of the bone. The problem in brow ptosis is mainly related to excess skin. The skin is very distensible, or elastic, but the aponeurotic layer is fibrous and is not. Advancing the fibrous layer doesn't do a good job of addressing the excess skin that is lying on top. That skin has got to be removed.

The dissection I usually use is in the subcutaneous plane, and there are a number of advantages to doing this. Number one, the nerves in the scalp are preserved. It also helps to minimize post-operative scalp numbness. Subcutaneous dissection also allow, for directly addressing the excess skin. In those individuals with promi-nent forehead wrinkles, the subcutaneous dissection also permits separation of these layers and smoothing of the wrinkles. Previous techniques relied on cutting the nerves supplied to the forehead muscles in order to paralyze them. This paralysis certainly resulted in eradication of the transverse creases, but it also resulted in a flat, lifeless forehead that lacked any expression.

"Well, that's no good," Marie offered. "What happens to the fa-cial expression? I mean, how do you make a point if your eyebrows don't move?"

You don't, I said. I also told Marie about a few other options:

· *The endoscopic technique.* This was devised to raise the brow with a minimum amount of scarring. Rather than the incision going completely across the scalp, the dissection is done through stab wounds using an endoscope. The stab wound is a small incision in the skin approximately one cen-timeter long. The endoscope is essentially a tube with a light and a dissecting apparatus on one end. It is used to accom-plish the dissection without the need for a long scar. The problem is that the procedure does not remove any of the ex-cess skin. It relies on advancing the forehead and tacking that either to a screw or a suture used to hold it in this elevated position. The problem I have is, once again, that you're pulling on the fibrous aponeurotic layer and not addressing the real problem, which is an excess of skin.

· *Botox.* Botox is short for botulism toxin A. It functions to eliminate skin wrinkles that are a result of muscle contractions. What Botox does is paralyze the muscle. I've used it a number of times, and it does in fact work well. I must admit, however, that I did have some fear about a patient having an allergic reaction, but to this point I have not had one. Nevertheless, the results obtained with Botox are transient, lasting two to three months, and therefore require reinjection to maintain the results. The areas injected are paralyzed and therefore lifeless. This does not affect overall forced expression because the paralysis is specific and localized.

Browlift Complications

Many of the possible complications with this procedure are those associated with surgery in general. They include bleeding and infection. Bleeding can lead to a hematoma formation; if that occurs, it will have to be drained. There are also complications that are specific to the procedure. They include:

· *Hyperpigmentation.* Usually results from residual blood whose breakdown products stain the skin. This can be avoided by the patient avoiding aspirin-containing medications and the surgeon adhering to strict hemostasis. Hemostasis is the act of stopping all bleeding.
· *Loss of skin.* Occurs when blood supply is interrupted. This is one of the drawbacks of the subcutaneous dissection. That

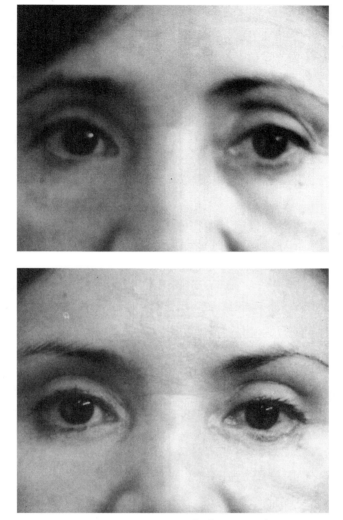

Figure 15: Preop and postop photos of a 47-year-old female browlift and upper lid blepharoplasty (eyelids).

is why this technique should be considered only when minimal temporal skin is excised.

· ***Hair loss.*** Is the result of loss of blood supply to the follicles, and the direct result of a scar. The surgeon must preserve

blood flow to the scalp, and zigzagging the scar can avoid noticeable bald spots.

- ***Nerve damage.*** Results from a technical error on the part of
  the surgeon. Dissection too deep in the temporal area of the
  scalp can injure cranial nerve seven, the facial nerve, leading
  to paralysis of the associated muscles.
- ***Hypertrophic scarring.*** Tension of the wound as a result of
  the skin excision can lead to a widened, thick scar. The tension can be minimized by limiting the amount of skin excised and by closing the wound in layers.
- ***Scalp numbness.*** With the coronal incision, some people
  also complain of persistent numbness of the scalp. This happens as a result of interruption of the ophthalmic nerve, and
  the numbness can be permanent. This can be a particular
  problem when the anterior hairline incision is used. Subcutaneous dissection can avoid this.

Marie was comfortable hearing about what could go wrong. She
was a survivor and, as I said before, she exuded confidence. She took
those possible complications in stride, choosing to focus on things
going well.

Blepharoplasty

As soon as I finished explaining the browlift procedure, Marie asked,
"What about my eyes?"

I told her that the eyes are fun to do. The results are predictable,
and most patients see an obvious improvement. The measurements
for the eyelid skin incision take place after the browlift is completed.
Care will have been taken to make certain that your eyebrows are
even and sit at the appropriate level. Once I'm sure of this, I'll measure the amount of skin to be excised from the upper eyelids and mark

the fatty deposits. I then inject the eyes with lidocaine, which contains epinephrine, and allow ten minutes for the epinephrine effect to occur. The epinephrine shrinks blood vessels and decreases bleeding. I'll then make an incision at the level of the eye fold, which helps to hide the incision. I'll also excise the fat in the upper lid and then close the whole area with a running suture. This will be removed on postoperative day five.

The lower lids require a little more work because I'm going to remove both skin and fat. The incision is made just under the lashes of the lower lid. I'll take care not to cut any of your eyelashes. Skin and muscle will be removed first, and then the fat. I'll close the wound with interrupted sutures of chromic catgut, which dissolve so they don't have to be removed.

Blepharoplasty Complications

Postoperatively, there are a number of things we need to watch for. If you know the warning signs, you can prevent these problems from becoming full-blown complications.

- *Corneal abrasaion.* During the operation, your corneas are protected by Lacri-Lube ointment and a protective contact shell. This is to prevent a corneal abrasion. A corneal abrasion feels as if you have something in your eye. If this happens, its only a nuisance and will heal within twenty-four hours, but it does require that you cover your eye and use a topical antibiotic.
- *Retrobulbar hematoma.* This is the most feared complication of eyelid surgery. A retrobulbar hematoma is bleeding behind the eye. It's a serious problem that can lead to blindness. An early sign of this problem is a feeling of fullness or pressure behind the eye. If one eye swells asymmetrically as

compared to the other eye, call me immediately. We need to address this.

- *Malpositioning of the eyelids.* This can take two forms: either an ectropion, which is a rolling outward of the margin of the eyelid, or an entropion, which is inversion of the lid. Immediately postoperative, I don't worry about these because swelling generally can cause either one. However, if the problem persists for more than three to four weeks, then we have to do something to correct it. That may require further surgery to relieve whatever tension may be affecting the eyelid.

- *Dry eye syndrome.* Can follow blepharoplasty and may be the result of incomplete closure of the eyelids. As a result, tears are not evenly distributed over the cornea and the eye can dry out, with subsequent irritation. This can be treated with eye drops and ointments, or may require further surgery to correct.

The Cost of Browlift and Blepharoplasty

The anesthesia for both procedures is approximately $700. If local anesthetics are used, the patient can save the price of anesthesia, being required to pay only for those supplies that are used. These procedures take two and a half to three hours in the operating room, which costs about $1,600. I charge $3,500 for the browlift and $5,000 for the eyes, and that's standard. The total is around $11,000. I know this sounds expensive, but it is truly an investment that will make you look good and feel good about yourself. The results of eyelid surgery are immediate, which makes it one of the most gratifying operations we perform.

And when I say the results are immediate, I mean it. The placement of the brow, removal of the lateral hooding, or overhang, and

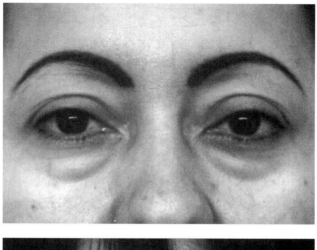

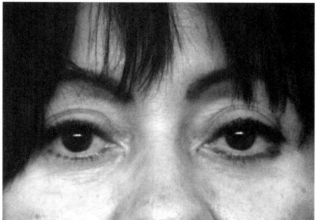

Figure 16: Lower lid blepharoplasty (eyelids) with removal of fat in a 44-year-old female.

the puffiness of the eyes is gone when the procedure is finished. There may then be some swelling, which is maximal at day three or four, but by day five after surgery the upper lid sutures are removed and you are socially presentable. Some people simply wear large sunglasses during this period and go about their regular activities.

By seven to ten days postoperative, you can wear makeup, and by three weeks postop this is all a memory.

Part Five

The Fifties

As we discussed in the previous section, women of color seem to age more slowly than Caucasian women. That observation, however, is somewhat misleading because we actually age in different ways. People of color age more in the forehead and eyes, while Caucasians age more in the lower face and neck. In addition, the sun more easily effects its damage on white skin. But many black people may eventually show signs of age in the lower face. For those women of color who do have jowling and wrinkling of the lower face and neck, a facelift may be appropriate.

It's important to remember, however, that having this surgery performed sooner rather than later usually brings about the best results. That is certainly a bias of mine, but I feel that if these problems are addressed before they are too bad, correcting them takes less time and money, the procedures can be smaller, and the results are more natural!

14

Facelift

THE FACELIFT PROCEDURE IS designed to address signs of aging in the lower face. I want to stress the *aging* aspect of that sentence. As I've said before, the major emphasis of rejuvenative surgery is to turn back the clock so that the outside physical appearance represents the vibrant person on the inside.

Ageless Alberta

Alberta was an elegant woman with a lyrical Spanish accent and light bronze skin. She said she was fifty-nine, though I suspected she was older. She was very proper and ladylike, which I associate with a previous generation. But perhaps her formal etiquette was the result of her Latin background. She looked good, though, and it was easy to see that in her younger life, she had been a very beautiful woman. I did not press her about her age. As I've said a million times, you're only as old as you feel. If she was shaving off a few years, her secret was safe with me. As far as I was concerned if she said she was fifty-nine, she was fifty-nine.

Even though most women of color age in the eyes and brows, Alberta had excess skin on her neck, and drooping jowls. She made it clear, though, that she didn't want her skin pulled so tight that she looked as though she were sitting on a cucumber. Actually, she said she didn't want to "look surprised," the cucumber is my description for the expression on an overly lifted face. That is probably how I would have described it to a patient who was more approachable, but Alberta's air of nobility made me feel that I should maintain some sense of professionalism.

We had our consultation in my office rather than the exam room because I felt she would be more at ease there. The room is formal, yet comfortable. I asked her to sit down in one of the leather chairs.

Our first order of business was to discuss medical history. This is particularly important when a patient is considering a facelift because it's an extensive procedure. In addition to the usual information, I pay special attention to the following factors:

- *Bleeding history.* It's important to know a patient's bleeding history because large flaps of skin are raised on the face during the surgery, and people who bleed easily can develop a hematoma, or collection of blood, with subsequent loss of skin.
- *Damage to facial nerves.* I need to know about any preexisting injury or weakness of the facial nerve so I can avoid further problems in the operating room. The facial nerve is crucial because it controls the muscles on the face that help us to talk and express our feelings.
- *Skin problems.* I need to know about skin problems, particularly cysts and abscess formations, which are localized collections of pus, and may be aggravated by this procedure.
- *Hair pattern.* Because the facelift incisions extend into the hair, I need to consider hair pattern so there won't be any bald spots in places that will be obvious after the surgery.

I found out everything I could about Alberta's past medical history. Although most aesthetic plastic surgery patients are healthy, I didn't want any surprises. Alberta's mother was one hundred and still doing well. Her father had passed away at the age of seventy-eight from prostate cancer. She had no children. Her only medical problem was glaucoma, and she was treating that with Timoptic and Dilocar. I really wasn't surprised that she was so healthy. Many of her relatives had lived to be well into their nineties or older, and you don't generally live that long unless you have good genes.

Even though Alberta seemed to be in good shape, I required her to have a chest X ray, an EKG, and laboratory work including a CBC and lytes prior to surgery. The CBC or Coulter Blood Counter was designed to evaluate the blood concentrations of cells, hemogloblin, and other blood contents, and the lytes (electrolytes) evaluate sodium and potassium in the blood. All her tests came back within normal limits. There were some irregularities of her EKG, but the cardiologist who evaluated them didn't think they should keep her from having the surgery.

After we discussed her medical history, I came around from behind my desk to examine her. Standing directly in front of Alberta, I placed my hands on her cheeks. I told her that the first thing I wanted to do was examine her skin. I needed to get some idea of its thickness and its elasticity. The elasticity is its ability to spring back. As we get older, our skin develops elastosis, which is loss of elastic tissue. As a result, it sags somewhat. Alberta had very high cheekbones, which was certainly to her benefit. People with flat cheekbones have a tendency to have lax skin and very prominent nasal labial folds. The nasal labial folds are the creases that run along the side of the nose and mouth. As we age, these creases becomes deeper.

"I have those," Alberta said. "We must do something about them, Doctor." She placed her hands on her cheeks and lifted up the lateral cheek skin, diminishing the depths of the nasal labial folds. "Like this," she said. "Can you do this?"

I smiled. I thought to myself, *I wish I had a nickel for every time I saw that.* Rejuvenation of the nasal labial fold area is probably one of the most difficult problems in plastic surgery. It's not as simple as just pulling up the skin. The tissue layers in the lips are compressed and well adhered to the layers above and below. However, those layers that make up the cheek tissue are loose and not so well adhered to the adjacent layers. Add gravity, atrophy of the subcutaneous fat, and elastosis of the skin, and you can see why the cheek skin begins to fall and drape over the compressed lip skin. The result is prominent nasal labial folds. A facelift can improve these folds somewhat, but it won't get rid of them altogether.

"What about collagen injections in the nasal labial folds?" she asked. "Would that get rid of these folds? I read something about collagen in a magazine."

I said that we could certainly do that, but it would not be permanent. Collagen reabsorbs over time, requiring repeated injections. This is not necessarily bad, though. If you don't like the result, there's solace in the fact that it won't last. In Alberta's case, though, I thought the best solution to her problem was a facelift. We could certainly get considerable improvement in the look of her nasal labial folds and, if needed, reserve collagen injections until afterward, when things had healed.

I then turned my attention to Alberta's jawline. It showed severe jowling, with skin and fat hanging below the level of the jawbone. This is a fairly common problem in older women. I explained that a facelift works well for correcting jowling, and I thought the procedure would give Alberta an excellent result.

Finally, I examined Alberta's neck. She had excess skin that hung down the midline like a turkey gobbler. This is also a very common problem. However, fixing it is much more complicated than just removing the excess skin.

I handed Alberta a mirror and asked her to look at the excess neck skin. In particular, I pointed to the vertical bands running up and down her neck in the midline. These lines represent the borders of the platysma muscle. The platysma muscle is one of the muscles of facial expression, and if you tense your neck, you can see it in action. When we're young, these muscles seem to overlap in the midline. With aging, the borders of the muscles separate, become lax and droopy as a result of gravity, and then become more prominent with time. In order to reestablish a youthful jawline, the edges of the platysma muscle need to be approximated and sewn. During the facelift, I pull at the lateral edges to place tension on this muscle, therefore getting rid of the turkey gobbler and these lines.

In an effort to be complete, I told Alberta that there are a number of other factors to consider when planning a facelift. The thickness of the neck and the prominence of the jawline contribute to the final look. Also important is the level of the hyoid bone in the neck. The hyoid bone is a small, horseshoe-shaped bone above the Adam's apple.

The muscles that form the angle of the neck attach to it. If the hyoid bone sits low in the neck, then the cervicomental angle, the angle the jaw makes with the neck, is obtuse and the jawline is not as attractive as when the hyoid bone sits high and forms a nice right angle. Although there was considerable neck skin, Alberta's hyoid bone sat relatively high in the neck, a clear indication that a facelift would provide a dramatic result that would be quite attractive.

The last things I wanted to examine were Alberta's earlobes and the character of her hairline. Both are important in the placement of incision. The hair is used to hide some of the incisions, but I also want to make sure that placement of an incision does not result in hair loss. This sometimes happens when the blood supply is compromised.

I also examined the earlobes for what is called pixie ear deformity. Pixie ear deformity occurs when the earlobes are pinned to the side of the face with the lobule attached to the cheek. If you're born with it, it's something that you tolerate, but it can be very bothersome if it's the result of the facelift procedure. Pixie ear deformity is

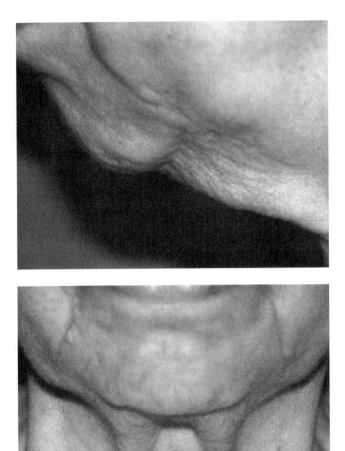

Figure 17: Turkey gobbler defect of the neck as a result of aging.

avoided by allowing for enough earlobe to fold under itself when closing the wound. Neither of these were going to be an issue for Alberta.

When the exam was complete, I told Alberta again that I believed she would get a good result from a facelift. But it's an extensive surgery, and I wanted to make sure she understood the procedure.

The Facelift Procedure

I prefer to use general anesthesia on patients during a facelift. There have been times, however, when I've used sedation or dissociative anesthesia with a medication called Propyphol. I supplement that with local anesthetics in some selected patients. In those patients who have had bad reactions, either an allergic reaction or severe nausea, to general anesthesia, this gives them another option, though the cost is higher. I also use this on patients who may have a health problem like asthma that makes intubation risky. I usually let healthy individuals choose the type of anesthesia they feel comfortable with—assuming the anesthesiologist agrees. I want the procedure to be safe, and I want the patient to be comfortable and have a pleasant experience.

You should arrive at the surgery center approximately one hour prior to the operation. At this time, you'll meet the anesthesiologist and the nurses. The anesthesiologist will go over your medical history. When you're done with the anesthesiologist's questions, I come in and mark the incision lines. Normally, the incision starts on the side of the head in the temporal scalp about 5 to 7 cm behind the hairline. It passes anteriorly, curving gently past the root of the ear, or helix, and then in front of the ear in the natural crease at the junction of the ear with the cheek skin. Staying in that crease, the incision proceeds posteriorly around the earlobe and up into the surface of the concha, which is the bowl of the ear, for about 2 to 3 mm. This insures that the final scar stays behind the earlobe and doesn't migrate onto the mastoid region behind the ear, where it can be seen. At the level of the tragus, which is the tonguelike projection of cartilage in front of the ear that hides the ear opening, the last leg of the incision turns posteriorly into the scalp. In those individuals who already have a high temporal line, or sideburn, a triangle of skin is cut out to prevent raising the hairline even further.

I also make certain that I address each individual's specific problem areas. The eyelids and the nasal labial folds are marked. Asymmetric areas, including those along the jawline, are identified and marked. If there is a severe turkey gobbler deformity of the neck, the submental incision in the platysma muscle separation is marked on the skin. At this time I also consider how to accomplish the best possible closure of the incisions.

These marks serve a number of purposes. They help to identify problem areas, they ensure that both sides of the face are dissected equally, and finally they ensure that the advancement of skin and subsequent skin excision are equal on both sides.

After the markings are complete, you are taken to the operating room, placed on your back on the operating room table, and your face and hair are washed with a Phisohex soap solution and painted with a Betadine paint solution. Whether or not you decide on general or local anesthesia, both sides of the face will be infiltrated with an anesthetic, most commonly lidocaine with epinephrine, to reduce the bleeding. I then wait approximately fifteen minutes for the epinephrine effect to occur before starting the procedure.

After you've been adequately prepped and draped, and the local has been given sufficient time to work, I'll start with your neck. I make an incision right under the chin, and deepithelize, or remove, the outer layer of skin adjacent to the incision so that at closure, I can overlap the two layers and prevent a crease under your chin. You've probably seen people with that crease under their chin that looks much like a witch's chin deformity. A witch's chin is the dimpling under the chin that makes the skin appear to overhang. I raise the skin flap in the neck and extend it laterally to the sternocleidomastoid muscles, the thick muscles on either side of the neck, and inferiorly to the level of the [Adam's apple]. I will then remove the fat in this area and take the opportunity to sew the edges of the platysma muscle together in the midline to get rid of those vertical bands in your neck.

Next, your head is turned to the side and I raise the skin flaps of the cheeks. The preoperative markings around the ears guide me as I make the incision. I address any bleeding as it happens, using electrocautery. Electrocautery is the use of an instrument that transmits electric current to stop blood vessels from bleeding. In an ideal situation, this part of the facelift would require simply removing the excess skin. In reality, however, that is rarely the case. Everyone has specific problems that need to be addressed. In Alberta's case, that was the platysma muscle. The platysma muscle is in a layer in the cheek called the submuscular aponeurotic system, or SMAS. Lifting the SMAS and the platysma muscle corrects the jowling and other deformities of the neck. Both the skin and SMAS are rotated superiorly and posteriorly by pulling the cheek skin toward the ear. The skin is then trimmed appropriately to inset into this incision. Prior to closure, a closed suction drain system is placed in the wound. This drain is there to remove any fluid or blood that accumulates under the flap during the initial postop period. It is removed the following morning. A bulky dressing is wrapped around your face and head to protect your incisions; this, too, will be removed the next morning.

Alberta nodded her approval. She knew I had done this procedure hundreds of times, and she appreciated my thorough explanation. Many patients don't want to know the details, but I think part of my job is to educate them as much as possible. I try to make sure that patients leave a consultation knowing as much about the procedure as they want to know.

Postoperative Care

I see you the morning after the procedure to remove the drains and dressings, and to make sure there are no problems. I first check to make sure there is no collection of blood under the skin flap. It is important that I monitor you for bleeding. Bleeding generally occurs within the first twelve hours after surgery. I also make sure that you are able to utilize your facial nerves; I check this by having you smile.

At five days postoperatively, I remove any sutures. I do this at this time to avoid any suture marks on the skin. The face is one place where you certainly do not want any suture marks. Swelling will be at its maximum at five to seven days postop. There will be numbness also, which may last for two to four weeks. Since you won't be able to feel anything, you will need to be careful about putting hot, cold, or sharp objects on your face. I ask my male patients not to shave.

I shouldn't need to say this, but you should *not* smoke either. The nicotine in smoke causes blood vessels to constrict, which can lead to loss of skin following surgery. This complication is a disaster no matter how you slice it. There is absolutely no question that cigarette smoking increases the risk of skin loss by about fifteen times. The short of it is, just don't do it. Don't smoke for two weeks prior to surgery and two weeks afterward.

I see you again at two weeks and three weeks postoperatively, These follow-up visits are to make sure that everything is progressing well. They are also a chance for me to give you a pep talk if you need it. This can sometimes be a period when patients become depressed. The surgery is over, but they haven't completely healed. Patients become anxious for it all to be over, and this leads to some depression. At three weeks postop, you'll begin to feel some itching, along with a pins-and-needles sensation in your cheeks. This is the result of the sensory nerves growing back into the skin. This will resolve with time, so bear with it.

I'll see you again at six weeks; by then you should be looking and feeling much better. We'll get together again at three months and six months postoperatively. We take your postoperative photographs at this last appointment. This is the best time to critically evaluate the results. You'll see excellent results by three weeks after the surgery, but I want to give you the full six months to heal before we critically evaluate the before and after photos to see if we've accomplished our goal.

Possible Complications

Having a facelift is a big, costly procedure that is not without risks. Patients who are considering this surgery need to be both physically and psychologically ready for it. Part of being psychologically ready is having realistic expectations. Otherwise, you're setting yourself up for failure—or at least disappointment.

Physically, we must be particularly careful of postoperative complications. They can lead to disastrous results if the proper care and attention aren't paid. Here are some of the potential problems that crop up with facelift procedures.

· **Hematomas.** Hematomas range from a small collection of blood that becomes apparent only after the swelling has gone down, to huge clots that threaten the survival of the facial skin flap. We need to do everything possible to prevent this complication. For two weeks prior to surgery, you need to stop all medications that interfere with the blood's ability to clot. This includes Vitamin E, aspirin, and aspirin-containing products. Many people are taking medications they don't even know contain aspirin; I'm talking about things like Midol, Excedrin, Alka-Seltzer, and Anacin. High blood pressure, coughing, and vomiting can also result in postoperative bleeding, and they need to be controlled. In reality, anything that increases venous or arterial pressure can be the culprit. Unfortunately, you can do everything exactly right and still get a hematoma. If you do get one, you'll start to notice it by feeling restless or uneasy. You'll just know that something isn't right. This feeling will then progress to pain isolated to one side of the face. The operative indicators here are *pain* and localized to *one side* of the face. Facelifts are anesthetic. They don't hurt despite the fact that for a few days you look like you were hit by a train. An isolated pain or asymmetric area of swelling should be considered a hematoma until proven otherwise. The treatment is to drain it, and that means removing a few sutures and evacuating the blood. This sounds like an extreme measure, but in the long run, it's smart and safe.

· ***Facial nerve injury.*** Injury to the facial nerve is devastating. The facial nerve controls the muscles of facial expression. If the nerves are hurt, the muscles that the nerves control become flaccid or weak. They simply stop working. The result can be a drooping of the involved area. If the injury is to the fibers around the mouth, one consequence may be drooling. Worse yet, the facial nerve is a cranial nerve and does not rejuvenate. If the surgeon cuts it, for all intents and purposes, the injury is permanent. That is a technical disaster that is best treated by complete avoidance, and believe me, that is exactly what I'll do. With the microsurgical techniques available today, I have to admit that the problem of flaccid facial muscles can often be addressed quite effectively. Nevertheless, no repair will be as good as the original. Remember my motto: the best way to treat a disease or problem is never to get it.

- *Loss of hair.* Sometimes patients lose hair in the surgical field, generally around scars. This is the result of decreased blood flow to the hair follicles or the scar itself. The solution is to plan scars away from hair-bearing areas that may be threatened.

- *Hyperpigmentation.* This generally manifests itself as a darkening of the skin due to the excess of breakdown products of blood. Any hematoma must be reabsorbed by the body, and this reabsorption process can result in staining of the skin. The best way to avoid this is to avoid hematoma formation, and to use a drain in the immediate postop period.

- *Hypertrophic scars.* These generally form behind the ears in a facelift. This is where the most tension is on the incision line, and tension is the cause of the thick scar. The scar can be revised secondarily or treated with a steroid medication, Kenalog.

- *Pain.* Facelifts are anesthetic—they don't hurt—and pain signifies that something else, either infection or bleeding, may be going on. This needs to be brought to the attention of your surgeon so that it can be addressed.

The Cost of a Facelift

Facelifts are among the most expensive plastic surgery procedures. The surgery takes about four hours to complete, and the total cost is around $12,000 to 14,000. This includes approximately $1,500 for the anesthesia, $2,000 for the surgical suite, and from $8,000 to $10,000 for the surgeon's fee. I know that sounds like a lot, but again, I think that it's a good deal. You will look years younger. And you can't put a price on looking and feeling good.

All in all, a facelift is a bargain.

As I knew from the beginning, Alberta was an excellent candidate for a facelift. Her result was fantastic, and the beauty that she clearly once was again declared her presence. I was happy for her. I liked the person she was.

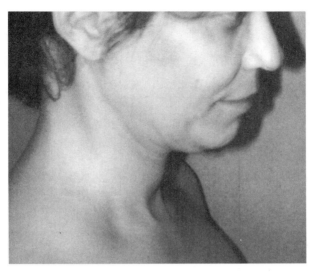

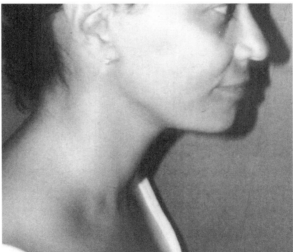

Figure 18: Facelift. Ideally the facelift procedure is designed to address aging and redundant skin in the lower third of the face. Here we have before and after photos of a 51-year-old female who underwent a standard cervico-facial lift.

-Part Six-

The Sixties and Beyond

Traditionally, this is the time when women are just beginning to think about addressing the effects of aging. However, there are major problems with waiting so long to address this issue. That's because when cosmetic surgery is put off until this stage of life, it involves larger procedures, larger costs, and higher morbidity rates. It also makes it harder to have natural-looking results. The physician must often take extreme measures to give patients the results they want. Therefore, they end up with that "done" look, which robs them of their clean, natural beauty.

From a plastic surgery standpoint, what's appropriate for women in their sixties (and above) are small touch-up procedures. The woman of color who has taken care of herself and followed my age-appropriate plastic surgery plan will need nothing more than small tucks behind the ears and around the neck and eyes. She might also consider small, localized areas of suction-assisted lipectomy to evacuate any unsightly bulges.

15

Touch-ups

LYDIA WAS A VERY pleasant woman in her sixties of Dutch descent who had married a black man. That is how I met her, through her husband. She had had a facelift a few years before but was unhappy with the result because, in her opinion, she looked "mean and unhappy," both of which, incidentally, were clearly not the case.

She did have one problem, though, and that is one common to facelift patients. While the facelift procedure addressed her jowling and neck, it did not address her aging mouth.

I pointed out to Lydia that as we age, gravity seems to effect more of its damage on the upper lip than the lower one. As a result, the upper lip becomes longer and thins out somewhat. The result is that in spite of the facelift procedure, the patient appears to be frowning.

Lydia's complaint is one that is quite common among those patients who have had facelifts. While the facelift procedure works well to rejuvenate the lower face and neck, it does nothing for the area around the mouth.

Procedures used to address this issue have included dermabrasion, skin peels, and various surgical procedures to reduce the length of the upper lip. The procedure which best addresses the aging mouth area is the Gullwing procedure.

And as Lydia pointed out, looking old and mean is worse than looking old.

· **The Gullwing procedure.** This procedure is based on the average measurements in young women and is designed to rejuvenate the oral area. The distance from the columella-lip angle (the attachment of the nose to the face in the midline) to the vermilion-cutaneous border (the white line of the upper lip where facial skin meets the mucosal skin of the lip) is 1.1 cm. With aging, this distance increases to greater than 2 cm. The result is a long lip that obscures the youthful 2 to 3 mm. show of the incisor (front) teeth. By excising a gullwing-shaped area of skin at the base of the nose to reduce this distance to 1.1 cm, the lip can be raised and "puckered" to give it a youthful look, and teeth show can be restored. Furthermore, by shortening the corners of the mouth by approximately ½ cm, the corners of the mouth can be shortened and the frown look that Lydia was referring to can be fixed.

Operative Procedure

In the preoperative holding area, the markings are made with the patient sitting upright and relaxed. An anesthetic gel is then rubbed on the skin, and after its effect has taken place, local anesthesia is injected and approximately ten minutes are allowed for the medicine to work. The skin is then excised according to the markings and the wounds closed so that the incisions are hidden in the crease just below the nose and at the angle of the mouth. The entire procedure is done under local anesthesia, with absolutely no discomfort, and the patient awake.

The Postoperative Period

Recovery takes much less time than one would expect. The first office visit for follow-up takes place at five days postop, and the sutures are removed at this time. (I will have called you on the phone on postop days one and two to make certain things are OK.)

After suture removal, you can wash your face normally and wear makeup. A follow-up visit is necessary at three weeks to evaluate progress, and at three months to take postop photos and compare results.

Advantages

This procedure allows for permanent rejuvenation of the lips without costly serial injections or the placement of foreign material to augment the lips.

Complications

The complications are those that go with any surgical procedure and really consist of bleeding. Both are avoided by strict adherence to surgical technique.

There is always the possibility of a thick, hypertrophic (widened) scar, and this is addressed with scar revision or injection of a steroid medicine called Kenalog to reduce the bulk of the scar.

Other Procedures for Rejuvenation of the Lips

- **Dermabrasion.** Used to smooth out the fine wrinkles around the mouth that are generally the result of smoking and sun damage.
- **Collagen injections.** Functions to augment the lips, giving them a fuller, more youthful appearance.
- **Lip augmentation.** Attempts to make lips fuller by injecting fat harvested from somewhere else on the body, or by using a Silastic strip (silicone with a

rubbery texture) placed under the skin to fill out the lip.

Costs

The Gullwing procedure is relatively inexpensive. It is done under local anesthesia and takes approximately one hour. The cost of the operating room and supplies is about $800, and the surgeon's fee is from $1,500 to $2,000, making the total from $2,300 to $2,800.

Lydia loved the idea of rejuvenating her lips without implanting some foreign material. She required no further information and signed up for the next available surgery date.

Her procedure went perfectly, within a week she was smiling, outgoing, and meeting new people without the fear of looking mean or angry. The smile that was hers was back.

16

The Successful Aging Beauty Solution

MY FUNDAMENTAL PHILOSOPHY IS that it's never too late to start doing the right thing. Throughout this book, I have attempted to emphasize that one of the major factors in cosmetic surgery is aging. Yet it's hard to speak of aging as a general term because one must specify the particular attributes of aging that are being considered. They can include skin elasticity, skin wrinkling, ptosis of the breasts, or the inability to sculpt the body with exercise. What can be said is that many aspects of aging are, in a sense, plastic. That is, they can be modified.

Here are my guidelines for controlling your own aging process. If you follow these simple steps, you'll always be beautiful because you will always feel in control.

1. **Consult your family physician.** Take control of your personal health. Find out how healthy you are and determine exactly what you can do to improve your overall well-being. Remember, effort and practice are required to maintain any function. For example, you can improve your lung capacity with exercise. You can improve your cardiac reserve by quitting smoking. You can make your skin healthier by avoiding the sun or wearing sunscreen. You can avoid

osteoporosis by taking calcium supplements and doing weightbearing exercises.

2. **Diet and nutrition.** The single most important dietary act you can engage in to age gracefully is to limit your caloric intake to less than 1,500 kilocarloies per day. Second, eliminate deep-fried foods and oils, including salad dressing. Third, reduce the amount of sugars you take in. Finally, take a dietary supplement that includes essential amino acids, vitamins, essential fatty acids, trace elements, and minerals.

3. **Skin care.** Always wash your face with a pH-balanced non-soap cleanser. Use a moisturizer that contains a sunscreen and antioxidants, including vitamins C, D, and E. Avoid the sun as much as possible. The best form of sunscreen is to wear protective clothing: long-sleeved shirts, long pants, and a hat.

4. **Exericse.** If you don't use your body, it atrophies and functions poorly. Engage regularly in a physical activity that challenges the heart and lungs. Do some form of weight-bearing exercise to strengthen bones. Use mental training, including reading and problem solving in math, on a regular basis to maintain cognitive function. Interact with other people and practice remembering things in order to preserve memory function.

5. **Count your blessings, not your troubles.** Develop the habit of looking on the good side of things. This will go a long way toward making you happy. The most powerful instrument at your disposal is your brain. Your reality is what your brain is focusing on at any appropriate time. Learn to control the focus of your mind. Usually, about 90 percent of what's going on in your life is good and no more than 10

percent is bad. The problem is, most of us focus on the bad 10 percent and ignore the good 90 percent. Learn to refocus on the positive 90 percent in your life. Count your blessings, not your troubles.

6. **Rejuvenative surgery.** Use small cosmetic surgery procedures, at age-appropriate times throughout your life, to ensure that your outer beauty mirrors the vibrant, beautiful person you are inside.

Index

abdomen, suction-assisted lipectomy and, 119, 123–24, 127, 129–31
abdominoplasty (tummy tucks), xi, 143–52
  age to consider, 9, 143
  cost of, 151
  duration of, 151
  possible complications in, 150–51
  postoperative period for, 149–52
  procedure for, 147–48
  scarring and, 49, 144, 146
abscesses, 66, 174
acetaminophen, 26
acetyl methoxycyrinate, 12
acne, 63, 69–72
actinic keratosis, 61
admission, 32
adolescence, see puberty
adrenocorticotrophic hormone (ACTH), 64
Adriamycin, 63
aesthetics, rhinoplasty and, 79
aesthetic surgeons, 15–17
  board certification of, 15–16
  collecting information on, 16–17
  consultations with, see consultations
  on day of surgery, 32–33
  rapport with, 17, 19–20, 22
  requesting alternatives from, 20
  selection of, 14–22, 102
  training of, 16
  and understanding your motives, 5–6
aesthetic surgery:
  cost of, xi, 8–9, 15, 21
  discussing risks, benefits, and complications of, 21
  goal of, 6
  morning of, 31–32
  motivation for seeking, 3–6
  popularity of, xi
  questions to ask yourself about, 5
  rejuvenative, 115, 117, 143, 173, 197
  as self-mutilation, 3–4
  tailoring it to individual, 90
  timing of, 8–9, 22
  as tool, 6–8
age, ages, aging, xii, 7–10, 73, 153
  abdominoplasty and, 9, 143

aesthetic surgical procedures appropriate to, 8–10
  in blacks vs. whites, 155, 159
  breast augmentation and, 9, 97, 100
  extrinsic, 59–60
  eyes and, 155–59, 171, 173, 183
  facelifts and, 171, 173, 175–78, 187
  graceful, 7
  guidelines for control of, 195–97
  intrinsic, chronologic, 59–60
  life expectancy and, 7
  markers of, 8
  mastopexy and, 9, 136, 138
  nutrition and, 11, 196
  physical appearance and, 8, 14, 156–57, 195, 197
  reduction mammoplasty and, 106
  scarring and, 49–50
  skin and, 12, 57–67, 70–71, 155–56, 158, 195–96
  suction-assisted lipectomy and, 9, 129
  touch-ups and, 189, 191–92
  variations in rates of, 8
  see also specific age groups
AIDS, 104–5
alar cartilages, 78–79, 87
alcohol, alcohol abuse, 38, 56, 155
  preoperative period and, 26–28
alpha and beta hydroxy acids, 70–71
Alzheimer's disease, 104–5
amputation, 107
androgens, 69
anemia, 24
anesthesia, anesthesiologists, 27
  abdominoplasty and, 147, 151
  blepharoplasty and, 168
  breast augmentation and, 97, 99, 101
  browlifts and, 161–62, 168
  cost of, 84–85, 101, 112, 130, 140, 151, 168, 179, 185
  on day of surgery, 32–33
  death rate associated with, 162
  dissociative, 179
  facelifts and, 179–80, 185
  general, 81, 86, 126–27, 161–62, 179–80

anesthesia, anesthesiologists (*cont.*)
  local, 81, 126–27, 161–62, 168,
    179–80, 192, 194
  mastopexy and, 138–40
  postoperative period and, 35–36, 38
  preoperative period and, 23, 31
  rhinoplasty and, 81–86
  suction-assisted lipectomy and,
    126–27, 130
  talking to, 31–32
  touch-ups and, 192, 194
anterior hairline incisions, 160–61, 166
antibacterial soaps, 28
antibiotics, 52, 127, 149, 167
  breast augmentation and, 97, 99
  mastopexy and, 139–40
  postoperative period and, 37, 40
  rhinoplasty and, 82–83, 86
antihistamines, 52
anti-inflammatory medications, 26
anti-malarial drugs, 63
antioxidants, 12, 196
  skin and, 62, 65, 68, 70–71
anxiety, xi–xii, 31, 36, 57, 182
Apollo Belvedere, 79
aponeurosis, 162–64
areolar tissue, 162
arms, 29, 60, 96, 129
aspirin, avoidance of, 26–27, 100, 104,
    164, 183–84
assets, protection of, 10–13
asthma, 104, 179
asymmetry, 101, 111
augmentations:
  of breasts, *see* breast augmentation
  of lips, 193–94
  of nose, 86–89
  rhinoplasty and, 81, 86–88
autoimmune disease, 91–92
average life span, 7
Avon skin products, 68–69

Bacitracin ointment, 40, 83, 99, 140
back, 129
bacteria, bacteria contamination, 29
  breast augmentation and, 94, 99
  mastopexy and, 139–40
  reduction mammoplasty and, 109
bandages, 40, 87, 110
  Ace, 51, 99, 139
  breast augmentation and, 99–100

mastopexy and, 139–40
basal cell carcinoma, 60
belly button (umbilicus):
  abdominoplasty and, 146–47, 150
  suction-assisted lipectomy and, 124
Bennelli lift (peri-areolar round block
    technique), 107, 135
Betadine solutions, 98, 109, 139, 147,
    162, 180
Big Macs, 10–11
biopsies, 65, 67
birth control pills, 61, 64, 122
bitemporal incisions, 161–62
blackheads, 66, 69
blemishes, 57, 69
Bleomycin, 63
blepharoplasty (eyes), xi, 159–60, 165–69
  age to consider, 9
  complications of, 167–68
  cost of, 168
  duration of, 168
  postoperative period for, 25, 165,
    167–69
  standard, 160
  transconjunctival, 160
blood, bleeding, blood vessels, 24, 48
  abdominoplasty and, 147, 150–51
  blepharoplasty and, 167–68
  breast augmentation and, 94, 96, 98,
    100
  browlifts and, 162–66
  facelifts and, 174–75, 177, 180–85
  hematomas and, 164, 167–68, 174–75,
    183–85
  mastopexy and, 138
  nicotine and, 28
  postoperative period and, 34–37
  preoperative period and, 26
  reduction mammoplasty and, 104, 109,
    111–12
  rhinoplasty and, 83–84, 87–88
  scarring and, 48
  skin and, 59–60, 65, 70
  suction-assisted lipectomy and, 122,
    127–30
  touch-ups and, 193
blood pressure, 28, 35
  high, 64, 184
blood tests, 86, 97, 122, 138, 175
  during preoperative period, 22, 24
blotchiness, xi–xii, 12, 57, 68

body temperature:
    postoperative period and, 35, 39
    skin and, 56, 59
bones, 73, 91, 177, 196
    rhinoplasty and, 77–79, 81, 83
    suction-assisted lipectomy and, 124
botulism toxin (Botox), 72, 164
bowels, 28, 40
bras, 100, 105, 109, 114
breast augmentation, xi, 29, 90–102
    age to consider, 9, 97, 100
    breast ptosis and, 95, 134–35, 137
    capsular contracture and, 93–94, 100–101
    complications in, 100–102
    cost of, 92, 101–102
    duration of, 95
    implant controversy and, 91–93
    incisions and, 95–98, 100
    mammograms and, 24
    muscle and, 94–96, 98
    procedure for, 98–100
    selecting surgeons for, 102
breast implants, see implants
breast lifts, see mastopexy
breast ptosis, 8–9, 133–37, 195
    breast augmentation and, 95, 134–35,
        137
    levels of, 133–36
    mastopexy and, 136–37, 139, 141
    pseudo-, 134–35
    reduction mammoplasty and, 106, 136
    solutions for, 134–36
breast reduction, see reduction mammo-
        plasty
breasts:
    cancer of, 104–105
    ideal size and shape of, 97, 102
    self-examination of, 104–105
breathing:
    postoperative period and, 37, 39
    rhinoplasty and, 80, 82–83, 85–89
    see also lungs
brow, aging and, 156, 158–59, 173, 187
browlifts, xi, 118, 156–66, 168–69
    age to consider, 9
    Botox and, 164
    complications of, 164–66
    cost of, 168
    duration of, 168
    endoscopic technique for, 163–64
    procedure for, 160–64

brow ptosis, 156, 159, 163
bruises, bruising, 26, 63, 129
        postoperative period and, 38–39, 42
buttocks, 129, 145

caffeine, 28
calcium, calcium supplements, 28, 196
calories, 10–11, 196
cancer, 11, 57
    of breasts, 104–105
    mammograms and, 25
    medications for, 63
    nutrition and, 11
    of prostate, 175
    of skin, 60, 62
cannulas, 122, 126–27, 129–30
capillary permeability, 48
capsular contracture, 93–94, 100–101
carbohydrates, 28
cardiologists, 25, 175
cartilage, 78–79, 81, 85–87, 179
Cesarean sections, 145–46
cheekbones, cheeks, 9
    facelifts and, 175–77, 179, 181, 183
chemical peels, 65, 71
chemicals, 59, 63
chest X rays, 25, 97, 175
children:
    scarring and, 43–47, 49–50, 53–54
    skin and, 57, 64
chin:
    facelifts and, 180
    rhinoplasty and, 77–79
chloride, 28
circumareolar incisions, 96–97
cleansing, see washing
clothing, 30, 39, 82
cocaine, 26–27
coffee, 28
cognitive function, 196
colchicine, 51–52
colds, 82
collagen, 41, 70, 83, 176, 193
    scarring and, 45, 48–49, 51–52
columella, 77–78
compression garments, 127, 129
concha, 179
constipation, 40
consultations, 5, 16–22
    abdominoplasty and, 145–47
    arriving early for, 18–19

consultations (*cont.*)
  and asking questions, 21–22
  blepharoplasty and, 166
  browlifts and, 157–66
  facelifts and, 174–78, 181
  fees for, 18, 22
  mastopexy and, 136–38
  and meeting aesthetic surgeons, 19–20
  physical examinations and, 20–21
  preoperative examinations and, 22
  preparing for, 18
  reduction mammoplasty and, 103–12
  rhinoplasty and, 76–82, 84–86
  second, 84
  suction-assisted lipectomy and, 117–28
contact lenses, 25, 31
corneal abrasion, 167
coronal incisions, 160–61, 166
corticosteroids, 50, 53, 67, 71
Coulter blood counts (CBCs), 24, 175
cranial-facial surgery, 14
cultural ideals, 79–80
cysts, 66, 69, 174

dark spots, 11, 60–64, 67, 70–71
death, 7, 162
de-epitheliazation, 109
deep pore cleansing, 70
dematosis papulsa nigra (DPN), 60, 66
dentures, 31
depression, 34, 182
  abdominoplasty and, 146, 151
dermabrasion:
  skin care and, 71–72
  touchups and, 191, 193
dermatitis, 29, 63
dermatolipodystrophy, 143, 146
dermatologists, 15
dermis, 59, 65, 67
deviated septum, 82
diabetes, 64, 104
Dial, 28
diastasis recti, 146, 152
Diburox, 29
diet, *see* nutrition
dietary supplements, 11, 196
Dilocar, 175
disrobing, 21
dorsal graft augmentation of the nose,
  86–89
dorsum, 80, 83, 86, 88
Dove Cleansing Bar, 68

drains:
  abdominoplasty and, 148–51
  facelifts and, 181–82, 184–85
  reduction mammoplasty and, 110, 112
driving, 29, 38
drooping, *see* ptosis
dry eye syndrome, 168

earlobes, 177–79
earrings, 30
ears:
  cleaning of, 28–29
  facelifts and, 179, 181, 185
  touch-ups and, 189
eating less, 10–11
ectropion, 168
edema, *see* swelling
ego, 5
elastosis, 158, 175–76
electrocardiograms (EKGs), 25, 35,
  97, 175
electrocautery, 98, 147, 181
electrolyte evaluations, 24, 175
emotions, 34, 38, 56, 58
employment, 5, 41
endocrine factors, 63–64
endoscopic browlifts, 163–64
entropion, 168
environment, 55–56, 59, 62, 66
epidermis, 65, 67, 70
epigastrium, 124
epinephrine, 127, 162, 167, 180
essential amino acids, 11, 196
essential fatty acids, 11, 196
estrogen, 61, 63–64
examination rooms, 105–106
exercise, xii, 8–9, 115, 195
  abdominoplasty and, 144–46, 150
  aging and, 195–96
  fat and, 13, 119
  postoperative period and, 41
  and protecting your assets, 13
  suction-assisted lipectomy and, 128
extrinsic aging, 59–60
eyebrows, 79, 156, 163, 166
eyeglasses, 31
eyelashes, 30, 160, 167
eyelids:
  aging and, 156
  blepharoplasty and, xi, 9, 25,
  159–60, 166–69
  browlifts and, 158–60

facelifts and, 180
malpositioning of, 168
eyes, 62, 72
  aging and, 155–59, 171, 173, 187
  browlifts and, 157–62, 169
  examinations of, 25
  touch-ups and, 189
  wrinkles around, 8–9, 156, 158
  see also blepharoplasty

face:
  browlifts and, 162–63
  nerves of, 174, 182, 184–85
  rhinoplasty and, 79–80, 86
  scarring on, 44, 50, 179, 185
  skin and, 57, 60–62, 68–69, 72,
    173–77, 179–83, 185
  suction-assisted lipectomy and, 129
facelifts, xi, 171, 173–87
  cost of, 84, 179, 183, 185–86
  duration of, 185
  nicotine and, 28
  possible complications of, 183–85
  postoperative period and, 181–83, 185
  procedure for, 179–81
  and selecting aesthetic surgeons, 15
  touch-ups and, 191
fainting, 38
false eyelashes, 30
family, 29, 91
family histories, 50, 91, 104, 122
  facelifts and, 174–75
  skin and, 59, 64
family physicians, 195
fascia, 144, 147–48
fat, fat cells, 28
  abdominoplasty and, 143–44, 146,
    148
  and aging around eyes, 155–56
  blepharoplasty and, 160, 167
  browlifts and, 159–60
  exercise and, 13, 119
  facelifts and, 176, 180–81
  mastopexy and, 137
  necrosis of, 111
  postoperative period and, 37
  skin and, 59
  storage of, 119
  subcutaneous, 121, 143, 145
  suction–assisted lipectomy and, 118–22,
    124–25, 129–30
  touch-ups and, 193–94

fatigue, 35, 38
fatty acids, 11, 63, 196
fibroblasts, 40, 48
fibroplasia stage phase of wound healing,
    48–49, 52
fibroplastic changes, 66–67
fifties:
  aesthetic surgical procedures appropriate
    in, 9–10, 171–87
  and EKGs and chest X rays, 25
  skin and, 57
fine lines:
  around eyes, 155–56
  skin care and, 67, 70–71
  see also wrinkles, wrinkling
fine-line scars, 45–46, 48–49
Fiorinal, 122
flexibility, 13, 48
fluids, 37
5-fluorouracil, 63
follicular responses and diseases, 66
follow-up examinations, 21, 99, 110, 128
  abdominoplasty and, 149–51
  facelifts and, 182–83
  mastopexy and, 140, 142
  postoperative period and, 39, 42
  preoperative period and, 23–25
  rhinoplasty and, 84, 87–89
  scarring and, 53–54
  touch-ups and, 192–93
forehead, 171
  browlifts and, 158, 160–64
  eyes and, 156, 158
forties:
  aesthetic surgical procedures appropriate
    in, 9, 153–69
  bodily changes in, xii
  mammograms and, 24
  skin care and, 67
Frankfurt horizontals, 77–78
freckles, 57, 60, 67
free radicals, 52, 62
fried foods, 11, 196
friends, 17, 29, 58, 119
  breast augmentation and, 91, 97
frontalis muscles, 156, 162

gender, 49, 60
genetics, 59, 61, 137, 175
getting up slowly, 37–38
glaucoma, 175
glucocorticoids, 63

gout, 51
grade 1 ptosis, 133–35
grade 2 ptosis, 134, 136
grade 3 ptosis, 134, 136
granulation tissue, 47–52
granulomatous changes, 66–67
greater trochanter (hip bone), 124
Gullwing procedure, 191–94
gynecologists, 15

hair, 29, 66
   browlifts and, 165–66
   facelifts and, 174, 185
   loss of, 165–66, 185
   preoperative period and, 29–30
hairline, 160–61, 166, 177, 179
hairpins, 30
hand surgery, 14
healing, 27–28, 113, 140, 167
   abdominoplasty and, 148, 150
   breast augmentation and, 94, 99–100
   facelifts and, 176, 182–83
   postoperative period and, 34, 40–42
   preoperative period and, 26–28
   rhinoplasty and, 83, 88
   skin and, 57, 59
   suction-assisted lipectomy and, 121, 128
   see also scars, scarring
health care reform, 15
health questionnaires, 18–19
heart, heart rates, 28, 35
   aging and, 195–96
heart disease, 57, 104, 153, 155
hematocrit, 138
hematomas, 164, 167–68, 174–75,
      183–85
hemochromatosis, 63
hemoglobin, 138, 175
hips, 119, 124, 145
homeostasis, 62
hormones, 120, 155
   breast ptosis and, 133, 137
   skin and, 63–64, 66, 69
hospitals:
   preoperative period and, 23, 30
   and selecting aesthetic surgeons,
      15–17
husbands, 5, 191
   abdominoplasty and, 145–46, 151
hydrogen peroxide, 40, 83
hydroquinone, 65, 67, 71
hygiene, 28–29

hyoid bone, 177
hyperpigmentation, 60–65, 68
   browlifts and, 160, 164
   causes of, 63–64
   facelifts and, 185
   skin care and, 12
hyperplasia, fat cells and, 119
hypertrophic scarring, 44–47, 49, 52–54
   breast ptosis and, 135
   browlifts and, 166
   facelifts and, 185
   reduction mammoplasty and, 112, 114
   touch-ups and, 193
hypertrophy, fat cells and, 119
hypopigmentation, 61, 66, 68
hysterectomies, 64

immune system, 52, 91–92
implants, 135–38
   breast augmentation and, 91–102
   breast ptosis and, 135–37
   controversy over, 91–93
   longevity of, 100
   mastopexy and, 137–38
   sizes of, 97
   textured, 93–94
inappropriate skin resection, 111
incisions, incision lines:
   abdominoplasty and, 147–49
   under arms, 96
   blepharoplasty and, 160, 166–67
   breast augmentation and, 95–98, 100
   browlifts and, 160–63, 166
   facelifts and, 177, 179–81, 185
   mastopexy and, 139–40
   postoperative period and, 39–41
   preoperative period and, 23
   reduction mammoplasty and, 107–108,
      110–14
   rhinoplasty and, 83, 88
   scarring and, 45
   touch-ups and, 192
infections, 82, 112, 130, 151, 164, 185
   breast augmentation and, 94, 99–100
   postoperative period and, 29, 39
   skin and, 55, 58
inflammatory phase of wound healing,
      47–52
inflammatory skin diseases, 63
inframammary fold, 133–35
inframammary incisions, 96, 98
ingrown hairs, 66

insurance, 25, 146, 152
    reduction mammoplasty and, 111–12
insurance verification forms, 19
intravenous (IV) lines, 33, 97, 139, 147
    rhinoplasty and, 82, 86
    suction-assisted lipectomy and, 126–27
intrinsic, chronologic aging, 59–60
itching, 29, 182–83

jawline, 176–77, 180
jewelry, 30
jowling, 9, 171, 173, 176, 181, 191

keloid scars, 44–47, 51, 53, 57, 112
    risk factors for, 49–50
Kenalog 40, 53, 114, 185, 193
keratinocyte cells, 58, 62, 65–66
kidney problems, 24, 155
knees, 126, 129–30
kojic acid, 71

Lacri-Lube ointment, 167
Langerhans cells, 58, 66
lasers, laser therapy, 51, 72
Lawyers Association of America, 92
legs, 129
lidocaine, 127, 162, 167, 180
life expectancy, 7
linea alba, 64
lipids, see fat, fat cells
lipodystrophy, 143, 145
liposuction, see suction-assisted lipectomy
lips, 77, 79, 176
    touch-ups and, 191–94
liver function tests, 24
lungs, 130, 153
    aging and, 195–96
    postoperative period and, 36, 39
    see also breathing

McDonald's, 11
McGann Company, 92–93
magnesium, 28
makeup, 30, 193
malanocyte cells, 58, 60–63, 65–66, 68, 71
malanosomes, 58
malnutrition, 28
mammograms, 24–25
marijuana, 26–27
mastoid region, 179
mastopexy (breast lifts), 100, 110–11,
    136–42

age to consider, 9, 136, 138
    cost of, 140
    duration of, 140
    postoperative care for, 139–40
    procedure for, 138–39
maturation phase of wound healing, 48,
    51, 53
maximum life potential, 7
mechanical injuries, 63
medical forms, 18–19
medical histories, 20, 24, 32, 64, 104,
    122, 138
    facelifts and, 174–75, 179
    rhinoplasty and, 82, 86
medical malpractice, 19
medications, 104, 122, 164
    abdominoplasty and, 147, 149
    facelifts and, 179, 183–84
    mastopexy and, 139–40
    postoperative period and, 24, 35,
        37–38, 40
    preoperative period and, 24, 31
    rhinoplasty and, 82–83, 86
    scarring and, 50–52
    skin and, 63, 65, 67, 69–72
    suction-assisted lipectomy and,
        126–27
    see also specific medications
melanin, 12, 59, 62–63, 65, 67, 71
    scarring and, 43, 51
melanocyte-stimulating hormone (MSH),
    63–64
melanomas, 60
melasma, 60–61
menopause, 64, 133
Mentor, 93
Merkel cells, 58, 66
metals, 63
methotrexate, 63
midline cartilage, 85–86
migraine headaches, 122
minerals, 11, 196
minimal scar techniques, 107
moisturizing, 56, 65, 68–70
mouth, 79, 191–94
    see also lips
Murine, 29
muscles, 13, 124, 156, 167
    abdominoplasty and, 144, 146–47
    breast augmentation and, 94–96, 98
    browlifts and, 158, 160, 162–64, 166
    facelifts and, 174, 176–77, 180–81, 184

narcotics, 26–27, 83, 99, 140, 149
    postoperative period and, 35, 37–38, 40
nasal labial folds, 175–76, 180
nasal obstructions, 85–89
nasal septal reconstruction, 25, 86–87
nasal turbinates, 82, 86
nasion, 77
neck, 9, 57, 60, 129, 189
    facelifts and, 171, 173, 176–78,
        180–81, 187, 191
Neosporin ointment, 40, 83, 99, 113, 140
nerves:
    browlifts and, 163, 166
    damage to, 130, 166
    facelifts and, 174, 182–85
nicotine, 28
nipple areolar complex, 64
    breast ptosis and, 135–36
    incisions around, 96–97
    reduction mammoplasty and, 107–108,
        110–11
nipples:
    breast augmentation and, 95–98,
        134–35
    breast ptosis and, 133–36
    devascularization of, 111
    malpositioning of, 111
    mastopexy and, 137, 139
    reduction mammoplasty and, 106–11
nitrous compounds, 64
nose, 25, 82, 85–89, 156
    augmentation of, 86–89
    browlifts and, 161
    touch-ups and, 192
nose surgery, see rhinoplasty
nostrils, 78–79, 81–83, 85–87, 89
numbness, 38, 166
nurses, 21, 32, 35, 139, 179
    abdominoplasty and, 147, 149
    breast augmentation and, 97–98
    suction-assisted lipectomy and, 126–27
nutrition, xii, 37, 52, 115, 119, 128, 138
    aging and, 11, 196
    alcohol consumption and, 26–29
    and eating less, 10–11
    preoperative period and, 26, 31
    and protecting your assets, 10–11
    skin and, 62, 69
nylon sutures, 99

Oil of Olay Cleansing Bar, 68
oils, 11, 196

operating rooms, 33
ophthalmic nerve, 166
optimism, 196–97
oral surgeons, 15
osteoporosis, 196
osteotomes, 81
otolaryngologists, 15
outpatient clinics, 15
oxygenation, 34

pain, 140, 149, 162
    breast augmentation and, 93,
        99–100
    facelifts and, 184–85
    medications for, see narcotics
    postoperative period and, 34–35,
        37–40
    reduction mammoplasty and, 103, 105,
        108, 114
    rhinoplasty and, 81, 83
pancreas, 28
papules, 60
parents:
    facelifts and, 174–75
    rhinoplasty and, 75–77, 82, 84–87
patience, 42
patient identification forms, 18–19
pectoralis muscle, 95–96, 98
pedicle, 107, 109–10
peri-areolar round block technique
        (Bennelli lift), 107, 135
periosteum, 162
peritoneum, 144
permeability, 48
personality, 58, 146, 151
pets, 38
pharmacologic agents, 63
phenol, 71
Phisoderm, 28
Phisohex soap solutions, 162, 180
photo-aging, 59–60, 195–96
photo-damaged skin, 70
photographs, 32, 42, 101, 178, 193
    abdominoplasty and, 150–52
    blepharoplasty and, 165, 169
    facelifts and, 183, 187
    mastopexy and, 140–41
    reduction mammoplasty and, 109–10,
        113
    rhinoplasty and, 78, 88–89
    suction-assisted lipectomy and, 121–26,
        131

phototransmission, 59
physical appearance, 4–5, 43, 115
    abdominoplasty and, 145, 151
    aging and, 8, 14, 156–57, 195, 197
    breast augmentation and, 91, 94–95, 97
    browlifts and, 163–64
    facelifts and, 173, 177, 183–86
    mastopexy and, 140–41
    postoperative period and, 38, 42
    rhinoplasty and, 80, 85–86
    skin and, 56–57
    suction-assisted lipectomy and, 117,
        123–24
    touch-ups and, 191, 194
physical examinations, 91
    abdominoplasty and, 143, 145–46
    consultations and, 20–21
    during preoperative period, 24–25
    rooms for, 105–106
physician-patient arbitration agreements,
    19
pigment, 57–58, 60–68, 71
    changes in, 66, 129
    see also hyperpigmentation; melanin
pixie ear deformity, 177–78
planning, 29–30
    to control timing and cost of aesthetic
        surgery, 8–9
    reduction mammoplasty and, 25,
        108–11
    see also preoperative period
plasticity, 8
plastic surgery, specialties in, 14
"Plastic Surgery for Women of Color," 3
platelets, 26
platysma muscle, 176–77, 180–81
postoperative period, 6, 21, 23–24, 29, 159
    abdominoplasty and, 149–52
    blepharoplasty and, 25, 165, 167–69
    breast augmentation and, 95, 99–101
    browlifts and, 163, 165
    from day three through day twenty-one,
        39–41
    facelifts and, 181–83, 185
    first few days of, 35–38
    immediately after surgery, 34–35
    mammograms and, 24–25
    mastopexy and, 139–42
    medications during, 24, 35, 37–38, 40
    one year after surgery, 42
    reduction mammoplasty and, 107–108,
        110, 112–13

rhinoplasty and, 83–84, 87–89
    suction-assisted lipectomy and, 118,
        128, 131
    things to expect during, 34–42
    three months after surgery, 42
    three weeks after surgery, 41–42
    touch-ups and, 192–93
postpuberty, skin care during, 70–72
potassium, 28
pregnancy, pregnancies, 115, 120
    abdominoplasty and, 144–46
    breast ptosis and, 133–34, 137
    skin and, 61, 64
preoperative holding areas, 32
preoperative period, 22–33, 141, 179
    abdominoplasty and, 147, 152
    blepharoplasty and, 165, 169
    breast augmentation and, 97–98,
        101
    browlifts and, 161, 165
    getting organized during, 29–30
    hygiene during, 28–29
    reduction mammoplasty and, 25,
        107–11, 113
    rhinoplasty and, 82, 84, 88–89
    scheduling visits during, 23–25
    substances to avoid during, 26–28
    suction-assisted lipectomy and, 125,
        130–31
    things to do during, 23–33
    and twenty-four hours before surgery,
        30–31
prepuberty, skin care during, 69
pressure garments, 51
Propyphol, 179
protection, skin and, 11–12, 55–56,
    66–68
protein, 31, 37
pseudo-ptosis, 134–35
psychiatric evaluations, 5
psychology, 3–4
ptosis:
    breast, see breast ptosis
    brow, 156, 159, 163
puberty, 103
    fat cells and, 119–20
    rhinoplasty and, 75–82, 85
    skin care during, 67, 69–70
puffiness, 155–59, 169
pulmonary embolisms, 36–37, 130
pulse oximeters, 35
pustules, 69

racial bigotry, 3–4
radiologists, 24–25
railroad track scars, 41
recommendations, 17
reconstructive surgery, 14
recovery rooms, 34–36, 83
recovery zones, 29–30
recreational drugs, 26–27
reduction mammoplasty (breast reduction),
    xi, 29, 103–14, 138, 141
  breast ptosis and, 106, 136
  complications of, 111–12
  cost of, 112
  duration of, 112
  preoperative period for, 25, 107–11, 113
  types of procedures for, 107
reproductive history, 143
Retin-A, 52, 69–70
retrobulbar hematomas, 167–68
rhinoplasty (nose surgery), xi–xii, 4, 9, 20,
    75–89
  cost of, 75, 84–85
  for nasal obstructions, 85–89
  scheduling date for, 84
  and selecting aesthetic surgeons, 15
rings, 30
Rudalgo Solutions, 12, 68–69

saddlebagging, 118–19
safety, 20, 32, 82, 104, 127, 138, 162
  breast augmentation and, 90, 92
  facelifts and, 179, 184
salad dressings, 11, 196
saline, 127
saline breast implants, 92, 99
scabs, 40–41, 83
scalp, 160–63, 166, 179
scalpels, 98, 147
scar revision surgery, 25
scars, scarring, xi–xii, 43–54, 57, 67, 69,
    71–72, 128
  abdominoplasty and, 49, 144, 146
  breast augmentation and, 93–94,
      96–97, 101
  breast ptosis and, 135–36
  browlifts and, 160–61, 163, 165–66
  face and, 44, 50, 179, 185
  how they are formed, 47–49
  mastopexy and, 137–39, 141
  postoperative period and, 40–42
  reduction mammoplasty and, 107–108,
      112, 114

rhinoplasty and, 83, 89
  solutions to, 50–53
  stretch marks and, 137, 144–46
  see also specific types of scars
Schamberg loop extractors, 70
screws, 163–64
second opinions, 18, 25
sedation, 162, 179
self-confidence, 153, 166
self-consciousness, 58, 63, 145
self-esteem, 75, 140–41
self-image, 5
self-suction, 148–49
septum, 25, 81–82, 85–87
seroma formation, 151
seventies, 60
sexuality, 42
significant others, 5–6, 91
Silastic strips, 193–94
silicone breast implants, 92
silicone gel pads, 51
sixties:
  aesthetic surgical procedures appropriate
      in, 10, 189–97
  bodily changes in, xii
  skin and, 57, 60
skeletal maturity, 73, 81, 91
skin, skin care, xi–xii, 11–12, 55–72, 195
  abdominoplasty and, 143–44, 146–49,
      151–52
  aging and, 12, 57–67, 70–71, 155–56,
      158, 195–96
  basics of, 67–69
  beauty regimen for, xii, 56–57
  blepharoplasty and, 160, 166–67
  breast augmentation and, 92, 95–99
  breast ptosis and, 134–36
  browlifts and, 158, 160–66
  cell types of, 58, 66
  contact dermatitis and, 29
  cysts and abscesses on, 174
  as excretory organ, 56
  eyes and, 155–56, 158
  face and, 57, 60–62, 68–69, 72,
      173–77, 179–83, 185
  loss of, 164–65
  mastopexy and, 137–39
  necrosis of, 111
  during postpuberty, 70–72
  during prepuberty, 69
  protection and, 11–12, 55–56, 66–68
  during puberty, 67, 69–70

reduction mammoplasty and, 107–10
rhinoplasty and, 78–79, 82, 87
as sense organ, 55–56
suction-assisted lipectomy and, 117,
122, 129–30
touch-ups and, 192, 194
see also scars, scarring; wrinkles,
wrinkling
skin color:
cells and, 58–60
scarring and, 49, 53–54
skin peels, 191
skin tags, 67
smoking, 28, 182, 193, 195
sniffers, 83
soda, 28
specialists, 15–16
splints, 83–84, 87–88
squamous cell carcinoma, 60
stair climbing, 38
standard blepharoplasty, 160
standard Wise pattern reduction, 107–109
state medical boards, 15–16
staying home, 39
Steri-strips, 99, 139–40
sternocleidomastoid muscles, 180
steroids, 127, 185, 193
scarring and, 50, 52–53
skin and, 65, 67, 71
stomach ulcers, 138
stratum corneum, 58–59
stress, 48, 57
preoperative period and, 23, 26, 31
stretch marks, 137, 144–46
subcutaneous fat, 121, 143, 145
subcutaneous tissue, 121, 143, 162–64,
166
submucosal turbinectomy bilaterally,
86–87
submuscular aponeurotic system (SMAS),
181
suction-assisted lipectomy (liposuction), xi,
117–32
age to consider, 9, 129
as body contour procedure, 121
comparisons between abdominoplasty
and, 143–45
complications of, 129–30
contour irregularities in, 129–30
cost of, 122, 130–32
oversuctioning in, 130
postoperative period for, 118, 128, 131

procedure for, 126–28
questions about, 120–26, 128–29
and selecting aesthetic surgeons, 15
touch-ups and, 189
sugar, sugars, 11, 37, 196
sun, 193
aging and, 59–60, 195–96
skin and, 12, 56, 59–61, 65–67, 70–71,
159–60
sunscreens, and, 12, 39, 65, 70, 195–96
suprasternal notch, 137
breast ptosis and, 133–34
reduction mammoplasty and, 106,
108
surgical centers, 16, 30, 32, 99, 179
abdominoplasty and, 147, 149
mastopexy and, 138–39
rhinoplasty and, 82, 84
suction-assisted lipectomy and, 126–27
sutures, 41, 84, 99, 110, 135, 139, 167
abdominoplasty and, 148–50
browlifts and, 163–64
facelifts and, 182, 184
touch-ups and, 192–93
sweating, 56–57
swelling, 29, 48, 127, 155
blepharoplasty and, 168–69
facelifts and, 182–84
postoperative period and, 38, 40, 42
rhinoplasty and, 88–89
Swiss Formula Body Lotion with Vitamin
E, 69

tea, 28
testosterone, 63
tetracycline, 52, 63, 69
thighs, 118–20, 123–24, 126–27,
129–31, 145
thirties, 13
aesthetic surgical procedures appropriate
in, 9, 115–52
bodily changes in, xii
skin and, 60, 67
thyroid disease, 155
Timoptic, 175
tip rhinoplasty, 86–87
tissue death, 130
touch-ups, 189, 191–94
advantages of, 193
complications of, 193
costs of, 194
postoperative period and, 192–93

trace elements, 11, 196
tragus, 179
transconjunctival blepharoplasty, 160
trauma, 63, 81
trichloracetic acid (TCA), 65, 71
tryosinase, 71
tummy tucks, *see* abdominoplasty
turgor, 129, 135, 137
turkey gobbler defect, 176–78, 180
twenties, 60
    aesthetic surgical procedures appropriate
        in, 9, 73–114
Tylenol, 26

ultrasonic liposuction, 119, 121–22, 130
ultraviolet radiation, 59–60, 66, 68
umbilicus, *see* belly button
under-eye bags, 155
upper eyelid surgery, 25
urinalyses, 24, 86, 97
urinary tract infections, 24
uterus, 144

vanity, 4
vegetable oils, 11
ventral hernias, 146, 151–52
Venus de Milo, 79–80
Vicryl sutures, 99
vitality, xii, 7
vitamins, 11
    A, 52, 68
    C, 68, 196
    D, 196
    E, 52, 68–69, 183–84, 196
    skin and, 62, 68

walking, 36–37
washing, 40, 113, 127, 140, 162, 180, 196
    abdominoplasty and, 147, 149
    breast augmentation and, 98, 100
    of ears, 28–29
    rhinoplasty and, 82–83
    skin and, 56, 68–70

weight, 11, 133, 145
    suction-assisted lipectomy and, 120–21,
        128
white blood cells, 48
whiteheads, 66, 69
wigs, 30
Wise pattern, 136
    mastopexy and, 138–39
    standard breast reduction and, 107–109
witch's chin, 180
women of color:
    author's experience with, xi
    comparisons between Caucasian women
        and, 10, 43, 49, 58–60, 66, 155, 159,
        171
    popularity of aesthetic surgery with,
        xi
wounds, 28, 40, 47, 140, 166–67
    abdominoplasty and, 148–51
    breast augmentation and, 98–99
    browlifts and, 163, 166
    facelifts and, 178, 181
    postoperative period and, 38, 40–41
    reduction mammoplasty and, 110
    suction-assisted lipectomy and, 121–22,
        126–28, 130
    see also scars, scarring
wrinkles, wrinkling, 60, 195
    browlifts and, 130, 158–61, 163–64,
        171, 193
    around eyes, 8–9, 156, 158
    skin care and, 11, 67, 70–72
    see also fine lines

Xeroform gauze, 99
xiphoid, 148
X rays, 25, 51, 53, 97, 175

youthful beauty, preservation of, xii, 7

Zest, 28
zigzag scars, 161
zinc, 52